Drawing Silk

Published by: Total Tai Chi
Fairview, NC 28730
USA

ISBN: 1-4196-6312-7
ISBN-13: 978-1419663123
Library of Congress Control Number: 2007901851

Visit www.booksurge.com to order additional copies.

Drawing Silk
Masters' Secrets for Successful Tai Chi Practice

Paul B. Gallagher

Total Tai Chi
Fairview, NC 28730
USA
2007

Drawing Silk

Table of Contents

Acknowledgements

First and foremost, I would like to acknowledge the generosity and support of my late parents. Even when I resigned from my doctorate study at a prestigious university to study Taiji full-time, they always fully encouraged me, though they perhaps did not quite understand...

I gratefully remember the snowy winter nights in Massachusetts when my Father would come to meet me around midnight at the cold and darkened Greyhound bus station, after my weekend commute back from studying Taiji in New York City. And, going through my Mother's possessions after she had passed away, I was amazed to find that she had saved all of the many flyers I had sent her about my classes and seminars, and often added her own notes and observations on the back of them.

Also, I am in tremendous debt to my teachers, Sophia Delza, T.T. Liang, B.P. Chan, Master Ken Cohen, and Sifu Ray Hayward for their great generosity in teaching and sharing their wealth of knowledge and skills with me. Also, to my very first martial arts teacher, Walter Mattson Sensei, master of Uechi Ryu Karate-do who gave me the spirit and attitude of persevering study. And to one Master Teacher, Jay Abraham, for giving me a whole new insight into how to teach—-and transforming my entire approach to teaching and writing.

I am grateful to my "T'ai Chi Brothers" Sifu Ray Hayward, Dr. John Myerson, and Master Tom Tunney for all the insights and good times we shared.

Thanks to Anne Griffin for typing and especially to Linda Pike who so ably helped with the final typing, formatting, and editing. Thanks to Becky Herdt for the beautiful cover design and her many helpful suggestions.

And to my many students and "Taiji Family" through the years who have shared the joys of learning, practice, and fun with me—the many studios we occupied over the years—from the funky "Violet Ray" to East Street, the Summer training at "The Willows," the cold winters on Deer Mountain, and the many festive banquets we shared. Many thanks also to Jessamyn (Ch'ing Mei) who made Deer Mountain possible, and to the intrepid "Old Timers" who helped build our Studio in Vermont during the frigid midwinter.

Thank you all!

"The spirit is at ease and the body tranquil, keep this always in mind. Remember, when one part moves, all parts must move; when one part is still, all parts are still...Internally, fortify your vital spirit; externally, appear peaceful and quiet. Step like a cat walking; move the intrinsic energy as though you are drawing silk threads from a cocoon. "

Wang Zong Yue, "Explication of the Use of Mind-Intent in Practicing the Thirteen Forms."

Preface to the Third Edition

The first two editions of *Drawing Silk* were written primarily as a resource for my personal students, as an adjunct to their practice.

Over time, I discovered that the book had gotten out to a wider audience and had been very well received. As the last copies of the second edition sold out, I began work on the present edition, which I hope will reach an even broader audience composed both of total beginners to the art of Taiji Quan, as well as to more experienced Players.

Notwithstanding the tremendous increase in the availability of Taiji instruction in the United States and the numerous books available, there are still only a relatively few books on Taiji Quan that contain the writings of the early Masters themselves. And, at a time when there are a great many proliferating "versions" of Taiji Quan, which are mere derivates of movement awareness or dance routines, the classical writings of the early Masters are an essential guide to correct practice and study.

This book is not a "how-to" manual for learning Taiji Quan. There simply is NO WAY of learning Taiji from a book, because you cannot see the flow or connection of movements from static images or verbal instructions. Video instruction is acceptable for learning the basics, or as an adjunct to learning from a teacher. But there is truly NO substitute for learning from a highly qualified teacher.

This book will give you the varying perspectives of a number of eminent Masters, as a guide to your study. The "Taoist Tales" at the end are actually a trilogy in themselves and illustrate some of the more esoteric aspects of practice. It is important to have a bit of insight into the total potential of the Taiji arts, since in current times the art has mostly been degraded to a gentle "relaxation exercise." There is so much more to Taiji than that!

You will find that *Drawing Silk* is a compendium of self-contained chapters, some of which duplicate information in other chapters, but from a slightly different focal perspective. Although chapters have been arranged in a sequence that seemed to present the material most efficiently, it is not necessary to read the book "from A to Z." You can pick up any chapter and read it independently, as your own interest or need dictates.

I hope the Masters' insights and the "Tales" give you some vision of the lifelong potential of dedicated practice following correct principles. Yes, you can indeed "retard old age and make Spring eternal," IF you practice correctly and perseveringly.

The first editions of this book used the older Wade-Giles transcription of Chinese characters. Here I use the worldwide standard *pinyin*, with the exception of those words that have already become standard use in English in their older transcription, such as Tao and Taoist. Also, the names of several well known Taiji Masters I write in Wade-Giles, since those names are a part of "common usage" among American Taiji Players. (Cheng Man Ch'ing, being an example.)

As for the word "Taiji," I often use it synonymously with "Taiji Quan," since most American students and Players call their art "Taiji." [Or, more commonly, Tai Chi. On the cover, I use "Tai Chi" for greater recognition by a majority of prospective readers.] Still, to be truly accurate, Taiji Quan refers only to the empty hand martial art section of the "Taiji System" just as Taiji Dao refers to Taiji Saber practice and Taiji Jian refers to the art of the Taiji Sword. Because most American students are primarily focused on the health and meditative aspects of Taiji Quan, and the broader aspects of cultivating personal harmony, my use of the word "Taiji" actually refers to the wider gamut of personal disciplines based on the Yin/Yang philosophy..

Finally, I have occasionally used s/he rather than alternate "he" and "she" or use only "he." S/he is becoming rather common in English usage, and I hope it leads to a smoother feel while reading.

To the many people who have been requesting this new edition for several years now, I want to say Thank You for your patience. As you know, books sometimes take on a life of their own, and that has certainly been the case here. I understand there has also been a considerable amount of web-searching on the part of people trying to find a used copy of *Drawing Silk*. One listing on E-bay even referred to *Drawing Silk* as a "lost classic!" Well, I am glad to say the new Third Edition has been "found" and I hope most sincerely that it truly benefits you in your study.

Introduction to the First Edition

This Deer Mountain Academy training manual is a compendium of articles I have written over the years to help students in their theoretical understanding Taiji Quan. Since Taiji Quan is an art that embraces not only the "practical" martial aspects, but is based on profound principles of philosophy, medicine, physics, and body dynamics, it is not enough to know the Forms alone. Practice of the physical aspects must be supplemented by study of its principles. Taiji is thus composed of both cultural (*wen*) and martial (*wu*) elements. Although no amount of theoretical study can substitute for unremitting practice of the Forms, practice of the Forms without correct principle will lead to a disheartening dead end. Once the basic physical functions have been mastered, deepening one's practice of Taiji Quan depends on the correct and subtle use of mental intention and imagery. The mental intent and imagery, in turn, depend on accurate comprehension of the Taiji Quan principles.

When I began my study of this art in 1966 there were only two books on Taiji Quan available in English. *Body and Mind in Harmony* by Sophia Delza was excellent in its treatment of fundamental principles and philosophy, but left out the more profound matters of meditative qualities and energy flow (which were reserved for her remarkable personal presence and "oral transmission"). And there was no mention of Taiji's defensive Applications. In both books there were some translations from the "*Taiji Quan Classics*" that inspired me by their depth and powerful imagery. I wanted to study these in more detail, but no literature was available in English. I decided to study Chinese and spent the next six years at the books in daily study. Upon meeting Master T.T. Liang in 1970, I had a rudimentary understanding of written Chinese and asked him if he could explicate some of the *Classics* for me. He very generously agreed and we spent the next several years reading many books and translating numerous texts that were published in 1974. This book was revised and expanded and published as *T'ai Chi Ch'uan for Health and Self Defense* (Random House, 1977). It was a great privilege to read the *Classics* and related books with Master Liang because reading them with understanding depends on:

1) knowledge of literary Chinese and numerous references to philosophy, medicine, and even martial arts "slang"; 2)practical knowledge of the application of the martial techniques; 3)sufficient command of English to translate the concepts adequately. Master Liang possesses each of these abilities in high degree. He explained to me that the *Classics* were written by the earlier Masters who had codified the fruits of their lifetime of practice into the terse and pithy phrases of literary Chinese. Only somebody who had embodied the principles through decades of training could fully elucidate their meaning in depth and detail. Nonetheless, even at a beginner's level, they describe the proper path of practice and set a clear direction for correct Taiji Quan.

During my period of intensive reading and study of the *Classics*, I became aware of the sizeable literature on Taiji available to Chinese readers. There are numerous books in modern Chinese that are fairly easy to read, as well as some in the literary language that are extraordinarily difficult. I translated some of the basic writings, which I have distributed to students throughout my years of teaching; but this is the first compendium of them all. Together with the numerous books now available in English, they can give sincere students an unerring direction toward fruitful study and enjoyable practice of this most wonderful and profound art.

The sections of this Manual are arranged in approximate order of importance from the elementary to the more advanced. Before each individual section, there will be a brief introduction detailing that section's significance and relevance to Taiji study as a whole.

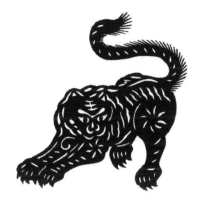

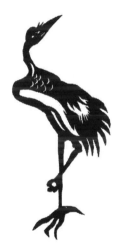

Chapter 1

Five Animal Frolics, Overview and "*Classics*"

Taiji Quan is an advanced level martial art, embodying numerous principles of balance, sensitivity, ability to sense and generate energy, to create and exploit an opponent's defective positions, etc. Traditionally, study of Taiji Quan presupposed or at least accompanied some knowledge of the so-called "external" martial arts, which fully stretch and condition the body, while teaching efficient use of power and speed. In Taiji Quan one who has already achieved some proficiency in these skills through strenuous training begins to internalize the training by moving more slowly through the formal movements, while emphasizing use of mental intention and imagery to guide the internal energy into its proper pathways for health and defensive use. It is presumed that by this time the student has already mastered the basics of correct posture, alignment, and body mechanics.

Since many American students come to Taiji as their first martial art or mind/body development study, I have taken the Five Animal Frolics as a prerequisite to other studies at the Academy. Created around 190 A.D. by Hua T'o, one of China's greatest physicians, the Frolics incorporate many of the principles of Taiji Quan, but in a more basic form. Unlike Taiji, which demands continuity of movement through the varied Forms for maximum benefits to health and energy flow, the Frolics can be practiced individually or sequentially as an invigorating system in their own right. Some of them, such as the Monkey and Tiger, are more vigorous and dynamic than the more subtle Taiji movements and stretch the body in more diverse ways.

This section includes a brief history of the Frolics, training principles, and the "Classics of the Five Animal Frolics" in an original translation.

Hua T'o's Five Animal Frolics — Overview and *"Classics"*

The famous Five Animal Frolics are the legacy of Hua T'o (110-207 A.D.), one of the great physicians of the Han Dynasty, and represent the only known remnants of his outstanding medical lore. They were transmitted to posterity by his disciple Wu Pu and to this day are a living testament to Hua T'o's dream of benefiting the health of all people. They are a gift of incalculable price.

In the *History of the Later Han Dynasty* , Hua T'o, speaking to his disciple Wu Pu says, "Man's body must have exercise, but it should never be done to the point of exhaustion. By moving about briskly, digestion is improved, the blood vessels are opened, and illnesses are prevented. It is like a used doorstep that never rots. As far as Tao Yin (bending and stretching exercises) is concerned, we have the bear's neck, the crane's twist, swaying the waist and moving the joints to promote long life. Now I have (created) an art called the Frolics of the Five Animals: the Tiger, the Deer, the Bear, the Monkey, and the Crane. It eliminates sickness, benefits the legs, and is also a form of Tao Yin. If you feel out of sorts, just practice one of my Frolics. A gentle sweat will exude, your complexion will become rosy; your body will feel light and you will want to eat."

Wu Pu practiced these exercises faithfully, training his body for perfect health. He lived to be over ninety years of age, still retaining acute hearing and clear eyesight, as well as strong teeth. His limbs were light and spry; his vital energy had not yet weakened.

The Five Animal Frolics, undergoing development and change throughout the passage of time, have now evolved into a number of schools, each with its particular characteristics and style. There are those that emphasize the imitation of animal movements; those that emphasize cultivation of inner *qi*; those that emphasize training the external; those emphasizing training the internal. Some emphasize developing hard energy, while others emphasize the cultivation of long life. Some emphasize combative techniques, etc. In any case, from the viewpoint of cultivating longevity, one should accentuate the training of *jing qi,* and *shen* (intrinsic energy, *qi*, and Spirit) when practicing the Five Animals, and give equal training to internal and external development. During practice one should attempt to achieve "tranquility within movement," controlling each movement by stillness of mind, use "suppleness within firmness," controlling the firm with the supple, finally reaching the stage where movement and tranquility are in equal balance, internal and external fuse into one, relaxation and tension can be equally applied, and firmness and suppleness assist each other.

The system of Five Animal Frolics taught at Total Tai Chi is mostly internal, emphasizing calm, relaxation, visualization (in some variations), and union of intent, breath, and movement.

The forms are graduated in degree of difficulty so that persons of any age or condition of health can practice. The variations can be practiced singly (depending on one's physical condition or time limitations) or sequentially as an invigorating complete exercise session.

The following points should be carefully observed during practice:

1)   **Movements must be rounded and lively.**
     In the Five Animals sequence most of the movements are curved, coiling, billowing, or twisting. The rounded movements are complete and smoothly joined. Even if the roundness is not obvious externally, during practice one must always maintain intent of circularity.

     "Lively" means that the movements are spirited and alert. Though the movements may be tranquil in attitude, they must never become lifeless, but always alert and energized.

2)   **Slow, steady, and reserved...**
     "Slow" means the leisurely pace of the movements. "Steady" means the solidity of the movements when qi has sunk. Only when you practice with leisurely motion and sinking of qi will your breath become soft, even, fine, and long. "Reserved" means that your use of energy in the Frolics

must not be manifest externally. It is concealed within and only you are aware of it.

3) Sequence of training:

The Crane and Bear are the most important and should be practiced first. The Crane provides a gentle warm up to the entire system, opening the gates of the spine and the major connecting meridians of the body. The Bear creates leg strength and develops energy in the Kidneys, the body's fundamental source of vitality. The Crane gently stretches the sinews; the Bear fortifies the bones. The Monkey is practiced next for suppleness and agility; the Deer for a long stretch to spine and legs; and the Tiger is the most external and dynamic. Some variations of the Crane and Bear should be practiced at each session. It is usually better to practice one or two variations of each animal for balance and variety rather than every variation of one animal and none of the others, if time is a limiting factor.

4) Coordinating breathing with movement...

Although some movements have definite breathing patterns, the most important requisite is to breathe naturally. The *Classics* say, "Forget the breath." When the forms have been mastered and the intent is right, you will probably find that the correct pattern is happening by itself. Above all never strain!

5) Speed and number of movements...

The movements should be neither too fast nor too slow; rapid jerky movement is to be avoided, as is excessive slowness leading to stagnation. When a movement has become slow and smooth, and the breath long and fine, one will have reached the correct standard. The number of repetitions can depend on one's level of health and proficiency. Sometimes good internal effects can come from doing one single movement many times, but in general, especially if one is doing the entire set, 9-12 repetitions of each is sufficient.

6) **"Beginning smooth, middle smooth, ending smooth..."**
Avoid imprecise or jerky beginnings and endings.

7) **General Advice:**
One should not practice when hungry, immediately after eating, when too tired, or when you are excited. Do not practice when emotionally upset or overly thoughtful. Before practicing, empty intestines and bladder; during practice make sure that clothing (especially belt) does not bind. Best times to practice are early morning and around sunset, but moments of leisure at any time my also be used. The practice place should have plenty of fresh air, but no heavy winds or atmospheric pollution. After practice you should not be too tired; always leave some reserve energy. A little bit of sweat (like gentle dew) is OK, but you should not sweat profusely, for this indicates strain.

8) **Practice must be accurate**
You should not allow distracted thoughts during practice. The beneficial effects of the Frolics—increasing bodily efficiency, correcting defects, and creating health cannot be achieved unless *jing* and *shen* are joined (vital energies and spirit are united and not squandered in distraction). Remember, within the movement there must be calmness and conscious control.

9) **Perseverance is essential**
The Five Animal Frolics are a type of *"nei gong"* (cultivation of internal energy); they are most efficacious in warding off disease and prolonging life. But they must be practiced for a period of time before yielding their full benefits. So you must have a trusting mind, a patient mind, a persevering mind. Training should proceed gradually and you should not try to learn everything at once. Practice time should be as consistent as possible from day to day to minimize missing training sessions.

Specific Points For Each Animal:
THE "FIVE ANIMAL CLASSIC"

1)   ## THE CRANE :
"must be light and soaring, calm and tranquil. Avoid heaviness and clumsiness."

The <u>Classic</u> says, *"The Crane is graceful, standing like a pine. It opens its wings and soars into the clouds. Spreading wings, it lands, poised on one leg: Its qi rises and sinks with no sense of heaviness."*

<u>Commentary:</u> The Crane is light and ethereal, and excels in flying. It is elegant and graceful, as if roaming the clouds or chasing the moon. While standing, it raises itself proudly like a lofty blue-green pine, standing eminently without moving. While practicing the Crane, one must have the far- reaching attitude of the Crane extending its wings through layered clouds without the slightest constraint. The attitude must be soft and supple, refined and leisurely. If the intent is heavy, the *qi* can easily stagnate and if the *qi* stagnates, the energy flow throughout the meridians cannot be harmonized.

2)   ## THE BEAR :
"must be ponderous, solid, and stable." Avoid lightness and airiness.

The <u>Classic</u> says, *"The Bear appears clumsy on the outside, but is alert and spirited within. Ponderous and solid, sunken and stable, but with lightness concealed internally. Its powerful flanks shake while moving and can be used to strike. Qi sinks to the <u>dan tian</u> (*center of energy below the navel) *and remains in the Middle Court."*

<u>Commentary:</u> The Bear appears clumsy, droopily shuffling along as though it had no bones. The Bear's nature appears ponderous and solid, sunken and stable, but conceals a

surprising lightness and agility. So in practicing one should not only express the Bear's attitude of ponderous stability, but its internal alertness and agility as well. Concentrate energy in the sides and waist, while allowing *qi* to sink to the lower *dan tian*. One can also retain concentration on the Ming Men point, (between the 2nd and 3rd lumbar vertebrae). After practicing for a long time, the kidneys and legs will be greatly strengthened and spleen and stomach harmonized.

3) **THE MONKEY:**

"must be quick-witted, alert, clever, and nimble." Avoid awkward, wooden movements.

The <u>Classic</u> says, *"The Monkey's mobile nature conceals a watchful calm. As agile and quick as a flash of lightning. He never remains still for long—stealing and offering the peach—how clever and startling!"*

<u>Commentary:</u> The Monkey's special ability is its fondness for movement. Climbing mountains, leaping across streams, and mounting trees to the topmost branches, its movements are extraordinarily spirited and lively. So if we want to imitate the Monkey's ability to move, we must especially train for tranquility in movement. This means training to be spirited and nimble externally while training the vital spirit to be peaceful and calm internally.

Practicing the Monkey's special movements of offering the fruit, one should pay particular attention to expressing its clever and mischievous attitude.

4) **THE DEER:**

"must be relaxed and extended, proudly erect." Avoid any sense of constraint.

The <u>Classic</u> says, *"The Deer is open and extended, its attitude relaxed, avoiding all restraint or forceful motion. It extends its body, leaps, and turns its head. Qi circulates to the tailbone and is cultivated in the sinews."*

Commentary: The Deer's body is open and pliable. While practicing the Deer, make sure your postures are released and comfortable. First of all, make your intention at ease (your energy and mind must not be tense). In movement, let there be not the slightest feeling of constraint; move freely and naturally, avoid forcing. Extending the body, leaping, and turning the head are all characteristic movements of the deer. While practicing the Deer, circulate the inner *qi* to the *wei lu* point (at the tip of the coccyx). Gradually, you will feel some sensation there. If you can circulate the *qi* through this point and into the Governing Vessel, in time you will develop very flexible sinews and bones.

5) **THE TIGER:**
"must be fearless, powerful, and awe-inspiring." Avoid timidity.

The Classic says, "*The Tiger's appearance is fierce and awesome; it is the king of animals. Externally strong, inwardly supple, deliberate and calculating. Moving like a whirlwind, tranquil like the Moon, pouncing, seizing and fighting its prey with invincible power.*"

Commentary: The Tiger is the king of animals; its attitude is fierce and awesome. While practicing the Tiger, you must express this by making the eyes spirited and the claws fierce. Its might is striking as it roars and screams, terrifying everyone. In using energy, be firm outside and supple within; while moving, be like the sudden onrush of a tempest; while still, be like the tranquil Moon of deep night, gradually attaining equal cultivation of movement and stillness, and mutual interplay of strength and suppleness. The Tiger's characteristic movements are pouncing and fighting its prey. By practicing these over a period of time you can greatly increase your strength.

My thanks to spirit friend and teacher Kao Han (Master Kenneth Cohen) for sharing this marvelous legacy of Hua T'o.

[To learn the "Frolics," you can do a web search. There are various teachers and videos available. The particular version of the Frolics described above taught by Paul Gallagher can be found on DVD at www.totaltaichi.com.]

Chapter 2

Reflections

This article was written in the early 1970's and contains elements of Sophia Delza's teaching of body dynamics, philosophy, and the psychological aspects of practicing the Taiji Quan form. Sophia Delza was one of the first Taiji Quan teachers in the United States who taught openly. She had studied in China in the late 1940's with Grandmaster Ma Yueh Liang, son in law of Wu Jian Quan, founder of the Wu Style. She passed away in 1996, at the age of 93 and was actively writing and teaching until three weeks before her passing.

My first Taiji Quan teacher, Sophia Delza was a master of the more subtle internal energy dynamics of Taiji Quan, as well as the psychic and spiritual changes a student progressed through in learning the art over a period of years. Studying with her was an ever-expanding experience of education and enlightenment in many areas untouched upon by the majority of Taiji teachers.

The next few pages summarize some of the essence of Sophia Delza's teaching—dealing with physiological, psychological, and philosophical aspects of practice.

[Readers who want to get right on to specific pointers for Solo Form practice might be advised to skip this chapter and return later.] But reading this chapter will be very rewarding in getting a larger vision of the overall effects of Taiji practice.

Some Reflections on the Art of Supreme Ultimate Boxing

Taiji Quan is a unique and beautiful meditative art, combining as it does physical, mental, and spiritual aspects to satisfy the needs of man on the three levels of his existence. In addition, Taiji Quan, because of its brilliantly conceived structure as an exercise, contains elements that stimulate and enrich man's philosophical, emotional, and aesthetic sensibilities. Translated literally the name means "Supreme Ultimate Fist" or, more freely "Supreme Ultimate Boxing." But the broader connotations of the title go far beyond this.

Beyond Taiji nothing can be conceived; nothing can be manifest. Hence the saying that Taiji (the Supreme Ultimate) is evolved from *Wu Ji* (the Non-Ultimate, the non-differentiated). On a more mundane level Taiji comes to signify the endless series of transformations of yin-yang-yin-yang in the Universe and in the mind and body of human beings. Taiji Quan is therefore an art that is based upon the principles of yin/yang interchange. Physically, it embodies alternate action (yang) and relaxation (yin) of each part of the body in turn; likewise the *qi* alternately flows toward the extremities of the body and returns to the *dan tian* .

In self-defense terms, any violent action (yang) directed toward the person is neutralized by retreating the body (yin) or twisting the waist, never presenting a firm or hard spot (yang) for the aggressive action to act upon. To return to our definition of the name Taiji Quan, it can be seen that in all its aspects this discipline is created according to the philosophy of yin and yang. Hence, the practitioner, through long experience with this art, eventually finds his interest and perceptions growing beyond the physical actions and into the realm of cosmology, deep study, and reflection upon the principles underlying the dynamic activity of the Universe itself.

The ancient sages of China who began experimenting with means to develop man's fullest potential perceived, as did the wise men of India who devised the techniques of Hatha Yoga, that unified and harmonious development of man's body and mind were essential if one was to realize the most profound possibilities of human life and activity. Throughout Chinese literature devoted to hygienic or meditative techniques one frequently encounters a dictum, terse, yet fraught with deep meaning that can be applied to many Chinese modes of exercise. *"Hsiu yang shen hsin"* (to improve or cultivate; to nourish; body and mind) implies that nothing should be overbalanced, that the condition of the body reflects upon the mind and vice-versa, and consequently that any means that one may employ to develop the self must take a unified development of body and mind into account. The creators of Taiji Quan as it evolved through the centuries, selecting from many existing techniques — innovating, creating, and refining — kept the goal of mind/body harmony in view as they devised the art that we presently refer to as Taiji Quan.

As a result of Taiji Quan's firm foundation upon the most profound and basic philosophical and cosmological principles of ancient China, performance of the exercise over a prolonged period enables the practitioner to acquire a very special and unique understanding and appreciation of Chinese philosophy and culture, not merely in a conceptual manner, but by experiencing the operation of these principles in one's own mind and body. Eventually one can bring an understanding of these principles to bear upon daily life as a whole, thus living every moment of daily life in full harmony with the Universe. It goes without saying that this final stage is not achieved without much perseverance, patience, and deep reflection.

In its insistence on maintaining perfect balance at all times, of pushing nothing too far, and of storing life energy carefully rather than dispersing it wastefully, Taiji Quan exemplifies especially the principles of Taoist philosophy. Indeed, tradition asserts that many of the progenitors of present-day Taiji Quan were Taoist sages, and ascribes to Zhang-San-Feng, a Taoist priest and immortal who dwelt on Wu Dang mountain, the creation of a prototypal Taiji Quan exercise, and the authorship of the primary *Taiji Quan Classic.* Unquestionably, anyone who has practiced the art will discover in Lao Tze's *Tao Te Ching* verbal expression of many principles learned intuitively in the course of Taiji Quan practice.

With regard to its physical characteristics as an exercise, the very first and most essential requisite of Taiji Quan is the relaxation of all unnecessary tension throughout the body. (Of course, merely standing or raising an arm involves some necessary and balanced muscle tensions). The reasons for this insistence upon "relaxation" are manifold. First, when the muscles surrounding the thoracic cavity are relaxed and false tensions disappear from the chest area, the diaphragm becomes able to move more freely and respiration becomes correspondingly deeper and smoother. One of the foremost maxims governing Taiji Quan practice is *"Qi chen dan tian"*—qi sinks to the *dan tian*. On a superficial level this indicates that the breathing must become slow and deep, controlled by movements of the diaphragm as if coming from the belly itself and not from the chest. More profoundly, the phrase indicates that the physical-psychic energies will eventually be developed and, in conjunction with deep respiration and concentration, will activate or "fill" the *dan tian* center—but this can only occur if the chest is relaxed and breathing is smooth.

Relaxation also implies the correct use of the body's energies without waste. As the student continues practice of the Taiji Quan Forms and comes to understand the subtle actions of joints and muscles that create the transitions from Form to Form, s/he becomes acutely sensitive to the use of muscular energies in the movements. In time this sensitivity can be applied in everyday life so that in any action one spontaneously employs just the right amount of energy in the correct proportions for any task at hand, thus decreasing fatigue and contributing to the possibility of a longer life.

Finally, relaxation of unnecessary external muscular tension aids the flow of blood to the organs. Taiji Quan not only seeks to nourish the body's external muscular structure, but, more importantly, seeks to ensure an unimpeded flow of blood through the vital organs. If external muscular activities are too vigorous, much of the body's blood supply will be called upon to serve the limbs and external muscles, while the vital organs of digestion, assimilation, and excretion (kidneys) will be given a reduced amount of blood. Meanwhile, the heart and lungs will be employed to a very high capacity. Taiji Quan, however, is a means of nourishing both the organs and the external muscular tissues simultaneously, and if movement is smoothly done, slowly and without tenseness, blood circulation to all parts of the body is free, balanced, and unhindered. The slowness of the actions also contributes to this effect, never causing the heartbeat or respiration to be unduly accelerated.

One of the most obvious features of the Taiji Quan movements, both to observers and performers, is the alternation of activity and rest for every part of the body. This is most evident, perhaps, in the movement of the legs. During the sequence of movements one leg is worked more forcefully by placing the greater portion of the body's weight upon it, while the other leg is straightened, thereby freeing it of weight and relaxing it. Throughout the sequence of actions there is a constant alternation of this working and relaxing. The hands also alternately wax and wane in forcefulness. A palm out-fingers up position changes to a movement in which the hand is withdrawn and the wrist unbent ("softened").

Throughout the 108 Forms and actions of Taiji Quan each portion of the body becomes fully activated and exercised, but because no one single part is ever in action continually in the same manner, one can complete the exercise with a feeling of repose rather than fatigue. From the physiological viewpoint this alternation of activity and rest does not create the accumulation of lactic acid that results when one muscle or muscle group is worked continually over a period of time, and therefore, there is no "oxygen debt" to be repaid, and no feeling of fatigue in the muscle tissues.

A particular advantage of Taiji Quan as an exercise is that the sequence of 108 movements (in the Yang or Wu Style "Long Solo Form") is so devised that the earlier movements demand less of the body than do those to come later. Thus, in the initial stages of the 25-minute exercise (done at beginner's tempo) the system becomes warmed up gradually, thereby greatly reducing the chances of any strain. Later, when the blood begins to circulate and the muscles have loosened up, more rigorous activity, such as high kicks or deep squatting positions, are demanded of the body. Likewise, in the process of learning the exercise sequence for the first time, the practitioner's body becomes gradually acclimated to the demands made upon it because the process of learning the 108 Forms extends over a period of many months. For this reason, even feeble or sick persons can begin their practice of Taiji Quan without fear of over-exertion and, in the course of time, can gradually and greatly improve their condition.

Unlike many forms of exercise and sports that merely use the body without regard to correct body action, Taiji Quan in every movement teaches the correct use of muscles and joints and can in time aid in the curing of postural and movement defects by showing the practitioner how to use the external body in the most efficient and graceful manner in all actions of daily life.

Beyond the level of physical technique in Taiji Quan lies the realm of mental discipline with its concomitant psychological and aesthetic factors. The student, as s/he progresses through the course of practice and learns the entire sequence of 108 Forms, may begin wondering why, if there are only 37 basic movements, must s/he perform all 108 actions? What is the purpose of the repetition of movement and of the variation in some of the repeated movements? Why not merely do the 37 movements and be done with it? As s/he continues performing the exercise, the student gradually perceives how the subtle variations that are so often expressed in a repeated movement have profound effects upon the feelings aroused in the mind during the practice of a round of Taiji Quan. Very frequently the repeated movements are so constructed that they enable the student to perceive the movement in a new light, to understand how the same movement can be generated from any one of several previous Forms, and thus, how Taiji Quan, as a whole, both philosophically and physically, can be said to consist of "one thousand changes, ten thousand transformations."

A repetition of a previously performed action may be done facing a new direction, thus affording the mind a kind of stimulation that would be lacking if the same Form were always directed toward the same point of the compass. (Sophia Delza in her advanced teaching also considered the different magnetic effects engendered in the body and energy flow by doing the Movements to the eight different directions). This sort of directional change in performing a Form already done also serves to keep the mind of the practitioner from straying. For if the mind wanders, one will almost inevitably do a repetition of a Form to the same direction that it was done previously, because the mind, like the body, all too easily falls prey to habit. But by constructing the sequence of Taiji Quan with such variations the creators of the art could ensure that practitioners would always find it necessary to maintain their concentration, to "stay alive" through every passing moment of the exercise because once a variant Form is incorrectly done, the succeeding Form cannot evolve from it easily, and the "flowing" sequence of movement becomes interrupted.

As the practitioner goes through an entire round of Taiji Quan movements, his/her mind is kept constantly enlivened as the old Forms evolve to something new and the new revolves again to the old, done in a slightly new manner. This arrangement contributes to the joy of performing the exercise and to the complete lack of boredom while doing it. For when the mind or body is about to become too fatigued with new actions, an old movement recurs, giving one a respite, and conversely, when the practitioner is about to become bored with the old actions, something totally new is called for in the sequence. This alternation of mental stimulation and mental repose is another most subtle use of yin and yang principles.

A second question often arises in the mind of the student after some months of practice. Why, if Taiji Quan is a means of attaining freedom in body and mind, must one constantly endeavor to perfect these movements, so demanding in stamina and concentration ? Why not just move about freely, move "spontaneously?" Can one attain "freedom" by constantly compelling oneself to conform to such precise standards as are embodied in the perfected forms and movements of Taiji Quan? Will this not create a sort of slavery instead of freedom?

Truly, freedom comes through discipline. For the diligent practitioner eventually comes to realize how the actions and indeed the entire gamut of daily Taiji Quan practice compel him to perceive his own weaknesses and to overcome them. The movements, though they may appear "effortless," are surely not perfected without effort, and going through an entire sequence of movement amidst the business of daily life demands that one be patient and persevering. Hence, during the process of learning this art, practicing it daily, and of perfecting it, one is made to confront one's deficiencies both mental (impatience, lack of concentration, etc.) and physical (weak legs, waist, etc.) and through gradual practice, without haste or anxiety, to overcome them. As the student looks back upon years of Taiji Quan study, s/he can see how the progressive elimination of physical and mental deficiencies through practice has indeed made one truly free, with mind and body vigorous and adroit.

The aesthetic benefits of Taiji Quan practice cannot be understood through words any more than one can perceive the joy of listening to a Bach fugue through hearing a lecture on counterpoint. But suffice it to say that when each Form is done smoothly and precisely with correct joint and muscular action and a calm yet concentrated mind, a "good feeling" arises from within, making one look forward joyfully to each day's round of practice. Though few current books on the art stress this factor, one who studies the writings of ancient masters of the Oriental martial arts will discover that the formal exercises (*katas* or "Forms") of many of these arts were devised not only as physical exercises or mental disciplines, but precisely to arouse within the participant these "good feelings" and thus to make one a peaceful and happy person.

The ultimate purpose of Taiji Quan practice is not only to exercise the external body, but to ensure an uninhibited flow of *qi* to every portion of the body. For, although the alternate contraction and relaxation of muscles and the movements of the diaphragm contribute to improving blood circulation, ancient Chinese medical treatises tell us that blood flow follows the flow of *qi*; hence, to ensure proper and unhindered flow of blood, the free circulation of *qi* must be achieved. Once the postures and the actions of joints and muscles have been mastered so that no unnecessary tension remains in the body and one can pass from one Form to the next with complete ease, free from any imbalance, then, through correct breathing and concentration, one can stimulate the *qi*, store it in the *dan tian,* and eventually cause it to flow throughout the entire body. When this stage is reached proper blood circulation will be assured, so that both the organs and the external musculature of the body will be fully nourished.

Furthermore, flow of *qi* is said to open the "psychic channels" in the body, and with this one enters into the realm of Taoist yogic practices. The books on Taoist yoga tell us that the spiritual energies cannot be activated in a weakened or clogged body, and that the first step toward awakening the spiritual energy is to clear out all toxic debris from one's tissues, blood, and "psychic channels" (equivalent to the major meridians of Acupuncture). When the flow of *qi* through all channels is free and uninhibited, then the practitioner may employ various techniques of concentration, breathing, and visualization to transmute the physical energies into pure *qi* and *qi* into spiritual energy. As in India yogic techniques, this energy is then employed to awaken the psychic center in the crown of the head, with all that this implies for the attainment of spiritual enlightenment.

Suffice it to say that Taiji Quan at its highest level can be a path of self-discipline leading to enlightenment. And it should be obvious that without a properly regulated (natural) way of life including good nutrition, sleep habits, and balanced lifestyle, that the pursuit of the highest goals of Taiji Quan would be quite futile.

As an art of self-defense, Taiji Quan stresses the absolute necessity of avoiding any direct confrontation with an opposing force. Rather, one learns to "root" himself firmly to the ground maintaining perfect balance at all time and yielding to an opposing force rather than meeting it directly. Practice of the Taiji Quan movement sequence develops this balance and rootedness and, since each posture has a "practical function" in warding off or counterattacking, one also learns many specific techniques of self-defense.

Diligent practice with many partners is required before one can delicately sense someone's energy, its force and direction and know intuitively and spontaneously how to neutralize the opposing force. One cannot learn "self defense" through words or concepts! But if one has developed a certain harmony within oneself, thereby becoming quiet, balanced, and unobtrusive, one may be far less prone to attract acts of violence and may be able to apply what the great master and founder of Aikido once called the only ultimate and foolproof method of "self-defense"—making the attacker your friend.

All of the above factors in combination make Taiji Quan a truly unique fine art of exercise and mediation, for it can be practiced on so many levels and for so many purposes. At whatever one's level of attainment, one can still discover new realms within the study of "Supreme Ultimate Boxing" and come to realize that the possibilities inherent in its practice are indeed infinite.

Chapter 3

Yang Ch'eng Fu's
Ten Essential Points

It has been traditional for masters to express the essence of their art, ripened after decades of practice, into a set of short aphorisms or sayings. Yang Cheng Fu (1883-1936) standardized the most prevalent current version of the Yang Style. These are Master Yang's famous "Ten Points" that can be considered the fundamental practice guides for Yang Style Taiji Quan. Master Cheng Man Ch'ing, one of Yang's most famous students, commented on these Ten Points in his well-known set of essays on Taiji Quan, "Master Cheng's Thirteen Chapters." These commentaries can be found in a translation by Prof. Doug Wile, *Master Cheng's Thirteen Chapters on T'ai Chi Ch'uan,* or in *Cheng Tze's Thirteen Treatises,* translated by Benjamin Lo and Martin Inn. Yang's Ten Points were originally oral teaching, later written down by Chen Wei Ming and published in 1925. Study and practice them well! I have appended a few personal comments enclosed in brackets.

Yang Ch'eng Fu: Ten Essential Points of Taiji Quan

1)   **Suspend the crown of the head lightly and alertly**

Preserving energy on the crown of the head (i.e. suspending the head) means that the head must be held perfectly erect, so that the vital spirit can reach the crown of the head. One must not use force; if one uses force, the muscles of the neck will be strained with the result that *qi* and blood will not be able to circulate freely. Rather, one must have a light and alert feeling. If the crown of the head is not suspended lightly and alertly, the vital spirit cannot be raised.

2)   **Let the chest be hollow and pluck up the back.**

"Hollowing the chest" means to let the chest be held in a bit [this means to release the chest gently inward—-NOT to "cave in" the chest] so the *qi* can sink to the *dan tian*. One must avoid forcing out the chest; if the chest is forcibly expanded, then the *qi* will accumulate in the chest with the result that the upper part of the body will be heavy and the lower part light; the heels will easily rise off the ground and one's root will be broken. "Plucking up the back" means that the *qi* must adhere to the back. If one can hollow the chest in the proper manner, then one can automatically pluck up the back; if one can pluck up the back, then energy can be issued from the spine so that one can be without match.

3)   **Relax the waist.**

The waist is the controlling axis of the entire body. If one can relax the waist, then the feet can develop rootedness and strength and one's stance can be secure. The interchange of substantial and insubstantial all derives from the rotation of the waist. Hence the *Classics* say, "The original source of the meaning of the Thirteen Postures is in the waist." If one's forms lack rootedness and strength, one must seek the cause in the legs and waist.

4) **(Clearly) differentiate the substantial and insubstantial.**

The number one principle of the art of Taiji Quan is to clearly differentiate the substantial and insubstantial. If the weight of the entire body is placed on the right foot, then the right foot is substantial and the left foot is insubstantial; when the weight of the entire body is placed on the left foot or leg, then the left foot is substantial and the right is insubstantial. If you have learned to clearly distinguish the substantial and insubstantial, then you can begin to move lightly and nimbly, without using the least bit of clumsy strength. If you cannot differentiate substantial and insubstantial, then your steps will be heavy and clumsy, your stance will be insecure, and you will easily fall under the control of an opponent.

5) **Sink the shoulders and let the elbows hang down loosely.**

Sinking the shoulders means that the shoulders must be relaxed and free and allowed to hang loosely. If you cannot relax them, they will begin to rise with the result that the *qi* will also rise and the entire body will be without real strength. Letting the elbows hang down loosely means to let them relax completely. [Simply imagine that your elbows are slightly heavy, pulled to the ground by the force of gravity.] If your elbows are held up your shoulders will be unable to sink and you will not be able to push an opponent far away. This will resemble the broken off energy of the external schools.

6) **Use mind-intent, do not use muscular force.**

The "Treatise on Taiji Quan" says, "The whole principle is to use mind intent and not muscular force." When you practice Taiji Quan, your entire body must be relaxed and open, so that you can release any stagnated energy in the sinews, bones, and blood vessels. After that you will be able to change your movements lightly and nimbly and turn your body at will. Some express doubts as to whether one can develop strength without using muscular force. Perhaps they do not realize that the human body contains pathways of energy just as the earth contains subterranean watercourses. If the watercourses are unobstructed, water will flow; if the body's energy channels are not closed off, the *qi* will reach every part of the body without hindrance.

If the entire body is full of stiff energy and the energy channels are clogged, then the blood and *qi* will become stagnant, your movements will be clumsy, and if even one hair is pulled, your entire body will be moved. If you do not use brute muscular force, but employ mind-intent, then wherever your mind is directed your *qi* will follow. In this way the *qi* and blood will flow freely and be conveyed to every part of the body without hindrance so that there is no stagnation or stoppage. If you practice this for a long period of time, you will acquire the genuine intrinsic energy of Taiji Quan. This is expressed in the "Treatise on Taiji Quan" as follows:

"When one has reached the ultimate point of softness and pliability, then one can reach the ultimate of strength and firmness."
One who has fully mastered the art of Taiji Quan has arms as soft as cotton externally, but with the weight of a heavy iron bar internally. One who practices an external art manifests his power when using it; when he is not exerting energy, he is liable to float and be unsteady. One can see that such a person's energy is external "floating energy." If one does not use mind-intent but uses only external muscular force, one can easily be trapped by an opponent and one's art will never reach a high level.

7) **The upper and lower parts of the body must move as an integrated whole.**

The meaning of the above phrase is expressed as follows in the "Taiji Quan Classic,"

"The energy is rooted in the feet, rises through the legs, is controlled by the waist, and is formed in the fingers. From the feet to the legs to the waist, everything must act as an integrated whole."

If the hand moves, the waist moves, the foot moves, the eyes and spiritual intent follow the movement—only this can be called "moving upper and lower parts of the body as an integrated whole." If even one part does not move, then the body's energy will be scattered and dispersed.

8)   **The internal and external must be in coordination.**

That which is developed in Taiji Quan is spirit-vitality. Therefore it is said, "The spirit is the leader; the body is the follower." If one's vital sprit can be raised, then every movement will be light and spirited. The Forms do not go beyond the principles of substantial and insubstantial, opening and closing. When one "opens," not only does a hand or foot extend, but the mind and intention must also extend outward. When one "closes," not only does a hand or foot come in toward the body, but the mind and intention must also draw inward. If you can perfectly coordinate the external movement with the internal intention, then gradually there will be no gap whatever between them.

9)   **Each Form (separate movement) must be joined to the next without interruption.**

The energy of the external martial arts [typified by Karate or Shaolin] is the brute muscular force of Later Heaven. Therefore it alternately waxes and wanes, is broken off and reconnected. When the old strength has been exhausted and the new is not yet developed (i.e. when one movement has finished and the next has not yet begun) one can very easily be controlled by an opponent. In Taiji Quan one uses mind-intent rather than muscular force. From beginning to end it continues fluidly without interruption. Completing a cycle and beginning again, it flows in an endless circle and is never exhausted. An early treatise says, "It is like a great river or the sea itself, flowing on endlessly without ceasing." It also says, "Mobilize the intrinsic energy as if you were drawing silk from a cocoon." [*The women who gathered silk from the cocoons of the silkworms had to carefully draw out each strand of silk with a precise and equal tension, so that the delicate strand would not break and the silk be lost.*] All of this refers to its continuity without break.

[I have found that the "drawing silk" principle has ramifications in almost every aspect of life. Have fun finding some for yourself!]

10) **In movement seek tranquility.**

The external arts are proficient in leaping and making forceful movements. They exhaust the breath and strength so that after practicing them one must pant for want of breath. Taiji Quan uses tranquility to control movement. Although one moves, one remains tranquil, so that in practicing the Forms, the more slowly one moves the better. When one moves slowly, the movement of the breath becomes long and deep, *qi* sinks to the *dan tian*, and the excessive tensing of the blood vessels is avoided. If the student examines each principle carefully and embodies it through unremitting practice, how can s/he fail to acquire the true meaning of all the above?

Chapter 4

Master Sung's
Twelve Guiding Principles

The Twelve Guiding Principles are from *Taiji Quan Xue* (*A Study of T'ai-Chi Chuan*) by Master J.J. Sung, a student of Professor Cheng in Taiwan. Master Sung's is one of the most complete treatments of the art in Chinese containing over 500 pages on history, philosophy, yin/yang interplay, classical writings and commentary, references to the *I Ching*, preparatory exercises, Taiji Quan Forms, and self-defense applications. One of the best books available, but still not translated into English. This version of the "Twelve Guiding Principles" follows Master Sung's very closely in translation, with a few additions of my own. While similar in some respects to Yang's Ten Points, they have a slightly different flavor and cover some additional areas. These Principles and "Yang's Ten Points" are essential knowledge for beginners, and even seasoned Taiji Players can benefit by reviewing them periodically.

J.J. Sung: Twelve Guiding Principles
of Taiji Quan

1) **In stepping, one must distinguish the Solid and the Empty.**

The first important point in Taiji Quan practice is learning how to distinguish the solidity and emptiness of the steps. The "Taiji Quan Classic" has already clearly pointed out, "The Solid and the Empty must be clearly distinguished. Each single part of the body has both a Solid and Empty aspect at any given time and the body in its entirety also has a Solid and an Empty aspect." From the very first Form, one must place the entire weight of the body on either of the legs and must let the sole of the foot adhere firmly to the ground, continuing thus until completing the final Form.

The Solidity and Emptiness of both legs is constantly interchanging. Only in this way can one acquire the marvelous effect of being light, relaxed, lively and nimble. A foot that adheres firmly to the ground, bearing the weight of the body and not moving is called solid; a foot adhering to the ground but not bearing weight and able to move is called empty. If both feet bear weight at the same time, one will commit the great error of double-weighting and will violate one of the fundamental principles of Taiji Quan and will also be unable to acquire the beneficial effects of this special kind of exercise.

2) **The movement of the hands must alternate activity and tranquility.**

In practicing Taiji Quan there are no movements in which the hands exert muscular force. As the hands form the movements, they always follow the shifts and turnings of the waist and legs. The hands never initiate movement on their own account. Indeed, if one sees an arm or hand moving independently, this is not in accordance with the principles of Taiji Quan. But the two hands, moving smoothly in the air with each movement joined together, create an alternation of activity and tranquility. Only by incorporating this interchange of activity and tranquility in Taiji Quan can the upper limbs and joints acquire the benefit of being completely relaxed. The "Treatise on Taiji Quan" says, "Taiji is the mainspring of motion and tranquility the mother of Yin and Yang. In motion they separate, in tranquility they fuse into one...Yin does not leave Yang; Yang does not leave Yin. They complement one another. To understand this is to understand intrinsic energy." If one practices the hand movements of Taiji Quan according to the principle of alternating activity and tranquility, then when one faces someone else, the movements will become an alternation of Solid and Empty. In motion the hands will be solid, in tranquility, they will be empty.

If both hands are empty, one will lose the effectiveness of the hand techniques and will be in a defective position. If both hands are solid, one is double-weighting and can easily be controlled by another. Therefore the "Treatise on Taiji Quan" says, "If you are double-weighted, you will be stagnant (unable to adapt readily and fluidly to circumstances). One often encounters those who, even after years of practice, cannot put their art to practical use and are subdued by others. This is because they have not yet understood the fault of double-weighting."

In performing the movements, one alternates the solidity and emptiness of arms and legs in opposition so that the energy of the leg on one side is connected with that of the arm on the other and vice-versa. In this way, one's center of gravity and balance will always be secure. Otherwise one will lose one's strong position and will easily fall under another's control.

3) **Completely relax the joints of the foot.**

The knee and ankle joints are the main pivot points in exercising the lower limbs. If one can rest them even for one brief moment, one should not pass up the opportunity. In this way one can develop them fully without exhausting them. In the practice of Taiji Quan the leg that supports the greater part of the body's weight is bent at the knee. The more empty leg, however, must also retain resilience at the knee and must not be straightened to the fullest extent (i.e. the rear leg in the "bow stance" and the forward leg in the "empty stance"). In each case the knee must be completely relaxed and no strength should be exerted to straighten the knee fully.

This is the principle expressed in the "Mental Elucidation of the Thirteen Forms…" "Seek straightness in the bent…" The ankle joint must also be completely relaxed so the sole of the foot can adhere to the ground firmly and solidly. In the "bow stance" the rear foot must not come off the ground and in the "empty stance" the forward foot must remain firmly placed and the toes must not be raised. [Most versions of Yang Style do raise the toes on the empty foot.]

4) **Relax the wrist and revolve the forearm.**

In the hand movements of Taiji Quan one must always relax the wrist joint completely, so that the bones of the forearm and hand can remain in perfect alignment (one smooth unbroken line from back of hand to forearm). In all of the hand movements of the entire sequence, with the exception of fists, Single Whip, and Beginning Form, one does not change the smooth unbroken line of hand and forearm. Therefore the flow of *qi* and blood to the palms and fingers can be abundant and the veins and vessels do not protrude from the back of the hand. But one must on no account use force to extend the fingers, nor should one allow them to bend lazily without extending energy. Again one must "Seek straightness in the bent." The spaces between the fingers are open naturally and comfortably. All of the above is included in the principle of relaxing the wrist. As the "Taiji Quan Classic" says, "Form is expressed in the fingers."

There is another important point relating to the relaxation of the wrist in Taiji Quan. In moving the hand forward or backward, in gathering and issuing energy, the wrist must follow the turning of the palm, the arm follows the turning of the wrist, each joint connected smoothly to the others while revolving. In this way one can acquire the softness and resilience essential to Taiji Quan practice. This way of revolving the forearm can in turn increase the effectiveness of relaxing the wrist. If one does not relax the wrist correctly, then the revolving of the forearm will not be beneficial.

5)   **Sink the shoulders and let the elbows hang down loosely.**

If the shoulders sink and elbows hang down loosely, it is proof that the joints of the upper limbs are relaxed. This is also one of the very first prerequisites of Taiji Quan practice. If a beginner has not yet acquired the proper feeling, he may try to force his shoulders to sink or his elbows to hang downward. In this case, he has clearly not yet understood how to relax and his rigid stiff postures will make this clear. This is because such a person has not understood the principle of using mind-intent rather than muscular exertion.

The changes of the hand techniques in Taiji Quan all rely upon mind-intent and not muscular exertion to issue and release energy. Sinking the shoulders and letting the elbows hang down in Taiji Quan bears no resemblance to forcing down the shoulders and covering the ribs with the elbows (defensive postures of some external styles). Therefore the "Taiji Quan Classic" says, "All of this relates to mind-intent within rather than external exertion." The intrinsic energy must not be visible from outside. One must relax every joint; if every joint is relaxed, then when one moves the hands, the shoulders will sink and the elbows will hang down spontaneously.

6)   Let the chest be hollow and tuck in the buttocks.

When one practices Taiji Quan one must let the chest be slightly hollowed inward and the buttocks tucked under. The purpose of hollowing the chest is to let the abdomen relax completely and the back to be held up erect, so the *qi* can sink deeply to the *dan tian*. The "Mental Elucidation of the Thirteen Forms" says, "When the abdomen is completely relaxed, then the *qi* can sink deeply and penetrate the bones...in pushing and pulling, moving back and forth, the *qi* adheres to the back." One holds the back erect so the *qi* can be gathered into the spine. However, to forcibly contract the chest or to push out the back like a camel's hump will cause tension throughout the upper body. This is altogether opposed to the principles of Taiji Quan practice.

The purpose of tucking in the buttocks is to make the lowest vertebrae plumb erect so that the *qi* can gather and the spirit can collect itself. Then the central axis of the body will be central and straight, allowing the body to be light and relaxed, lively and nimble. As the "Song of the Substance and Function of the Thirteen Forms" says, "When the lowest vertebrae are plumb erect, the vital spirit rises to the top of the head. When the top of the head is held as if suspended from above, the entire body feels light and spirited." If one practices Taiji Quan and disregards the above rules, one will deviate from the fundamental principles of the art.

7)   Relax the neck, hold up the head.

"Empty" (completely relaxed) means that one uses no muscular force to straighten it (the neck). Nor does one allow it to collapse so the head is crooked. Rather, one uses the neck's own natural elasticity to suspend and centralize the head so that the head is perfectly erect and centered. This is a very important point in the practice of Taiji Quan. It is as if a thread held up the crown of the head so that the head in turn settles down lightly upon the shoulders without pulling away from them upwards or pressing them downwards. One just allows the head and neck to be relaxed and natural. In this way the head and upper body will be erect and centered so as to follow the movement of the waist. In addition, the passage of nerve impulses through the neck and the circulation of blood and fluids will be enhanced. The responsiveness of the nerves will be sharpened so that one can develop the alertness and agility to use the movements in self-defense. As the "Song of the Substance and Function of the Thirteen Forms" says, "When the top of the head is held as if suspended from above, the entire body feels light and spirited."

8) **Let the eyes look inward.**

When your head and neck are erect and centered, it is inevitable that your eyes will gaze straight forward. Gazing straight forward means that the eyes and spirit do not concentrate upon a single point but are open and receptive to the entire surroundings. The eyes and face are completely relaxed. The phrase in the "Taiji Quan Classic," "The spirit should be concentrated within" is based on the principle of turning the gaze inward. On the contrary, if you gaze outward, focusing your eyes concentratedly on external things, your vital spirit will stream outward and be scattered. Your reactions will no longer be quick and spirited and you will find it very difficult to acquire the true effectiveness of the Taiji Quan techniques. If you can achieve this turning the gaze inward (i.e. not looking intently at anything in particular), you will be able to gaze forward at the expanse before you, looking at nothing but seeing everything.

9) *Qi* sinks to the *dan tian*.

In practicing Taiji Quan the ability to concentrate the spirit and collect the *qi* is given special importance. Sinking the *qi* to the *dan tian* is the first principle of concentrating the spirit and gathering the *qi*. When you inhale, you use mind-intent to direct the *qi* downwards; then the lower abdomen feels light and relaxed. Soon you feel that the inner organs are gradually relaxing and sinking. At this time the place in the lower abdomen that feels full and rounded is the *dan tian*. As the "Taiji Quan Classic" says, "The *qi* should be stimulated." To speak of this is easy enough, but it is not so easy to accomplish it.

One often sees those who have practiced for years without any result. Although in theory this involves change deep within the body, one can verify it externally with one glance. One whose *qi* has really sunk to the *dan tian* will have a completely relaxed upper abdomen, while the lower belly will be rounded out and full. It has nothing to do with distending the lower belly with forcible breaths in or out. The feeling of letting the *qi* sink must be maintained throughout the entire round of Taiji Quan movements. In Taiji Quan practice sinking the *qi* is of primary importance because only after the *qi* has sunk can one begin to mobilize the movements of the body with the *qi*. After a long period of practice the True Qi will overflow the *dan tian* and will circulate to every part of the body so that the movements will be fluid and smoothly connected like floating clouds or running waters.

10) Circular Exercise

The movements of Taiji Quan all advance in a circular line. When the forward and backward movements of Taiji Quan are connected, large or small circles are formed. The "Treatise on Taiji Quan" says, "Stand like a poised scale; move like a cartwheel." The "Mental Elucidation" says, "The mind and *qi* must interchange in a spirited manner so as to develop a rounded and lively tendency. This is called the transformation of Solid and Empty." Therefore, if the hand movements in Taiji Quan are not rounded, they cannot be lively. If one's movements can be rounded out, then they will be lively and agile and if every action can be rounded then one can retain a superior position at all times.

If the body moves actively like a cartwheel and the hands follow the body movements, then the movements will naturally be circular. In this way the Forms turning left and right, rounded and lively, will be like shooting stars, and the entire body, interchanging the Solid and Empty smoothly and continuously, will become comfortable, open, light, and spirited. Then one can discover the potential of each movement to neutralize opposing forces.

11) **Movements must be smoothly connected.**

When one begins the practice of Taiji Quan, each movement must be thoroughly mastered before one can proceed to the next. In this way, as learning progresses, each succeeding Form can be smoothly connected to the preceding without any breaks or discontinuity. Then the entire sequence can be performed continuously and fluidly. As the "Taiji Quan Classic" says, "It is like a great river or the sea, flowing on endlessly...there should be neither deficiency nor excess, neither hollows nor projections, neither severance nor splice." All of this indicates the necessity of connecting each movement smoothly to the preceding and following.

In connecting the movements one must remember four fundamental principles: light, slow, even, and correct proportion. Moreover, each movement must be circular as described previously. Only in this way can they be correctly joined without break. If they are not light, it will be difficult to make them rounded, lively and smooth. If they are not slow, one will find it difficult to acquire the relaxed and rounded feeling. If they are too slow, however, the *qi* can easily stagnate and the movements lose continuity. If the movements are even, then they will appear smoothly connected, and if the proportions of all the movements are correct, this proves that all of the above principles have been observed.

12) Each movement must involve the entire body.

Each Form and movement in Taiji Quan involves the entire body internally and externally, mobilizing the muscles, bones, joints, and sinews, and energizing the internal organs (the Zang and Fu, compact and hollow organs). The principle of Taiji Quan practice is that the movements of the limbs must harmonize with the movements of the entire body, rising and sinking, moving forward and backward, left and right. As the "Taiji Quan Classic" says, "In every movement, the entire body must be light and spirited and all of its parts must be connected like a string of pearls... where there is up, there must be down; where there is (a movement) forward, there must be a movement rearward; where there is left, there must be right." This is the basic rule of moving in Taiji Quan.

The "Mental Elucidation of the Thirteen Forms" says, "Always remember, if one part moves, all parts move; if one part remains still, all parts remain still." As the "Song of the Substance and Function of the Thirteen Forms" says, "Whether bending, stretching, opening, or closing, let it take its natural way." This means that when one part stretches out, then the entire body seems to open outward; when one part contracts, the entire body pulls inward. When the correct method of body movement has been perfected to a high degree of skill, your breathing will also naturally accord with the movements.

There is no absolutely fixed method of breathing in Taiji Quan. Each Form will naturally demand a certain type of breathing. However as a general rule, one inhales when moving inward or upward, exhales when moving outward or downward. But it would be a great error to forcibly attempt to co-ordinate breath with movement because this would violate the fundamental principles of naturalness in Taiji Quan and would cause the movements to lose their rounded and lively quality and the *qi* and blood to become congested and stagnant.

Chapter 5

"Master Gao's"
Ten Essential Points

This set of Ten Points was written by a former dweller on "Deer Mountain" in a quiet corner of Vermont, after friends and students prevailed upon him to leave some vestiges of his experience. Some of the Points concern preliminaries for practice of the Solo Form, such as the leg strength and body alignment; others deal with mental attitudes. I have found them useful both as a guide to teaching and in my own personal practice.

Ten Essential Points for Taiji Quan

1) **ATTITUDE** toward progress must be relaxed, devoid of ego aggrandizement, non-linear. Progress in Taiji Quan study, like the yin / yang spiral, is paradoxical, exposing ever deeper levels of ourselves. By "trying" too hard, we lose the essence of spontaneous growth and development. In practice we must listen to our *qi* with relaxed unhurried mind and perfectly unclouded awareness.

2) **STRENGTH** in legs and lower spine, best attained through standing meditation, holding basic Taiji Quan forms, or special exercises. Only if your legs are sufficiently strong and back straight can your steps be firm, agile, and controlled, with clear distinction of solid and empty. Most beginners lack sufficient leg strength to make smooth, even steps, so auxiliary exercises are very beneficial (provided they conform to Taiji principles).

3) **CORRECT ALIGNMENT**, inner and outer. Attention must be given to carefully aligning your shoulders and hips, nose and lower *dan tian*, ears and shoulders. Standing postures are good to create awareness of alignment without the added mental input from movement and Forms. Inner alignment involves sensitivity to the lower, middle, and upper *dan tian*, as well as free circulation of breath and *qi* through organs and meridians. Faulty alignments will block this flow and cause stagnation of breath (caused by off-centered alignment of shoulders and hips) or *qi* (caused by meridians that are compressed).

4) **STRETCHING** and meridian opening to release mechanical blocks. The Taiji form, using mind to visualize and guide *qi* through the body is a very subtle form of *nei gong* (cultivation of internal energy). Beginning students often have mechanical misalignments that cause the flow of energy in the "meridians" (channels of *qi* used by Acupuncture) to be blocked, so it is often very beneficial

to do initial stretching exercises and *qi* development movements to maximize beneficial effects from the Taiji form.

[You can find DVD's with instruction of these special exercises on totaltaichi.com.]

5) SOLID AND EMPTY steps must be clearly differentiated, and can best be learned through repetitive exercises of stepping with proper joint-flow-release. When doing your Taiji Solo Form, sequentially—gently and easily—release weight from your heel, to knee, to hip of the leg that is becoming unweighted. This is a great secret of practice.

6) STEADY LEVEL of your Taiji Solo Form, without dipping or rising. Your hips, shoulders, and eyes maintain the same level to develop endurance and strength in the legs and a quiet spirit It is difficult to maintain "meditative" centeredness of mind if the eye-line and horizon are continually rising and falling. Sophia Delza used to say, "Be like the horizon of the sea, not like a cork bobbing on the waves."

7) AN IMAGE of Application or purpose in each movement is essential for moving the *qi*—it must be learned, then felt, and finally forgotten (*wu wei*), as the *qi* flows more and more spontaneously through each movement. The Image creates the open pathway; later full relaxation and alert spirit will cause the *qi* to circulate without such specific directives.

8) "MERIDAN" PATHWAYS should be known, so *qi* flow can more accurately be directed through the proper energetic channels.
   You might want to find a good chart of the Acupuncture "Meridians" just to get a feel for where these channels are. But it is NOT necessary, even counter-productive, to try to force energy to flow in these channels—just be aware of them.

Later, simply visualizing the inner breath moving through the meridians will cause *qi* to flow; thus promoting health and vitality in the internal organs.

9) **GOOD NUTRITION.** Since we are trying to build *qi* (bio-electrical life-energy), heavily processed food, food that has been stored a long time, and heavily chemicalized food, will only cause stagnation in the body. Food must be light in quality, fresh, and look healthy (have a radiant aura). You must develop sensitivity as to whether or not your food has *qi*. Strict vegetarianism is not essential, but a simple diet consisting of grains, vegetables, nuts, seeds, seasonal fruits, and small amounts of clean animal food (especially poultry and fish), balanced according to principles of hot / cold and seasonal factors, is optimal for producing *qi* and reducing stagnation from excess food or feces in the digestive organs that will deaden *qi* flow.

[See www.totaltaichi.com for an entire program devoted to balancing nutrition and other life factors. "Your Master Key to Perfect Health."]

10) **POETIC SENSE** of the Grand Taiji. All of our efforts to "practice" the Form, develop *qi*, health, defensive ability, etc. will be incomplete if we cannot open our selves to the great ocean of *qi* that surrounds us at every moment. Passing clouds, flowing waters, the majestic turns and spirals of celestial bodies, the procession of day and night and the Four Seasons—all these are the Grand Taiji Quan Form going on around us at each moment. After mastering points 1-9, forget the entire business and let the Grand Taiji of the universe play itself through "your" movements. Ego is gone; effort disappears; you are open and empty, allowing Tao to flow through your central axis or Taiji ridgepole, the spine, and four limbs. Like a bronze bell hanging from a mountain temple, you resonate in perfect harmony with the *qi* of everything around you.

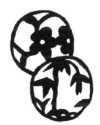

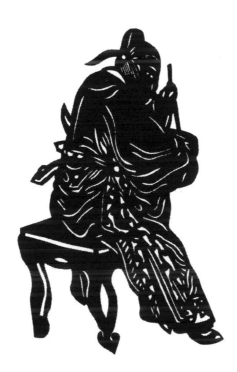

Chapter 6

"Taiji Quan by the Numbers"

The same Player from the wooded hill, inspired by the teachings of the late B.P. Chan, who often used number images in his vivid presentation of principles, compiled this set of nine steps to "Taiji Immortality." The mnemonic images are often good to meditate on before engaging in the Form so they may resonate in the deeper levels of your mind during practice. It is best to select any one item and focus on that just before practicing, so your training in the Solo Form reflects the principle involved. When you have progressed through all nine after a period of weeks or months, return to number one again and begin the cycle anew.

When you can apply all of these "numbers" consistently in your daily practice, you will surely be a "Taiji Immortal."

B.P. Chan taught in New York City for a number of years and was a marvelous synthesizer of Internal martial arts principles in his teaching.

Taiji Quan by the Numbers

"Taiji Quan by the numbers" is a series of mnemonic devices to help in remembering and actualizing Taiji Quan principles in your practice. Some of them are from the teaching of various masters; many of them are original. The approach "by the numbers" is inspired by the classical Chinese literary principle of "saying much with little", or using the minimum number of words to express ideas of great depth and with manifold ramifications.

1) **The One, unbroken unity**, the *Wu Ji* (the undifferentiated Oneness of the Universe), before Yin and Yang have spun themselves off into the Taiji (opposite yet complementary forces). In practice this refers to a standing meditative posture such as "Holding the Moon" or "Holding the One," letting the arms embrace an imaginary ball while the feet are placed slightly more than shoulder width apart. (All specific instructions must be from competent teachers). In Lao Tze's *Tao Te Ching*, Chapter 10, we find a reference to "embracing the Unity." This is the unified, still and focused mind, the "Full Moon" of our True Nature, the beginning and end of all Taiji Quan practice.

2) **Two is Yin and Yang**—up/down; in out; forward/backward; and the multiple dualities of the Taiji in practice and in life. We cultivate this awareness by using the "Raise Hands and Step Up" Form of Yang Taiji Quan as a standing meditative pose to develop sensitivity to the varying yin/yang balances of all parts of the body. Interchanging this pose from right to left teaches light "empty stepping," and the changing yin/yang balance of arms, legs, feet, and hands.

3) **Three Heavies and Three Lights**: Using this Principle you can create relaxation with alert awareness throughout your body. (Heavy means sunk and deeply relaxed and has no connotations of stiffness or immobility). Keep your knees heavy (slightly bent), elbows heavy (to relax shoulders and

chest), and tip of lower spine heavy (like the plumb on the end of a line). Keep the top of head light, (lifted effortlessly without strain), fingertips light, and eyes light (no fixed or strained expression). The light head and fingertips counterbalance the heavy coccyx and elbows.

There are also Three Methods:
Foot Method (proper stance),
Body Method (correct use of the waist), and
Hand Method (application of hand techniques).
In practice, first adjust your feet, then body, and lastly hands, building up your Form like a tree or house on a solid foundation.

Finally the Three Levels: Keep your "Eyes level, shoulders level, hips level." No bobbing up and down during the Form.

4)   **The Four "F's":**
        Form
        Function
        Feeling
        Forgetting

First you learn the sequence of movements, correct transitions, etc. This is Form.

Then you must learn the proper (defensive) Applications of the Form to understand the purposefulness of the movements in depth, as well as how to image the flow of *qi* in each Form. This is learning the Function.

From long practice of Form and Function, you will develop a Feeling for the flow and use of energy in each movement, and the *qi* will begin to flow spontaneously, following the Feeling.

When your spirit can vitalize the movements without specific mental intention or imagery, you will realize that Taiji is moving you; you are completely "empty," yet aware. As the ancient verse says, "Without form, without shape, entire body thoroughly empty." This is the stage of "Forgetting."

The "Four F's" can have tremendous ramifications in every area of your practice.

First, the Four F's come about naturally in your initial process of learning Taiji Quan. Once you have learned the Solo Form, then you can strategically use the Four F's in your daily practice.

On a day when you are scattered and unfocused, you can emphasize Form in your practice. That will keep you grounded and centered.

Emphasizing Function will give your Solo Form a greater aliveness and intensity on a day you feel lazy or lethargic.

Focusing on Feeling lets you concentrate on the flow of energy with a sensation of ease and contemplative awareness. This is good for a time when you are stressed out.

And Forgetting comes as a gift when you have so completely integrated all the other F's that your Solo Form seems to do itself.

Master Liang used to call this stage of practice, "going to Heaven without spending one dime."

5)   **The Five Hearts:**
> Two soles of feet,
> Two centers of the palms
> And the heart itself

All are important centers of energy and must act in coordination and harmony and be joined by subtle flows of energy.

6) **The Six Harmonies**:
Three Outer Harmonies — shoulders align with hips; elbows with knees; hands with feet.
Three Inner Harmonies —
The mind harmonizes with the Intention (the mental focus which directs each movement); Intention harmonizes with *qi; qi* harmonizes with strength.

During practice it is especially important to be aware of these Six Harmonies at all times.

7) **The Seven "Rounded Places"** of the upper body (especially in such movements as the Yang Style "Ward Off" Form, or the "Holding the One" mentioned above).
1)From spine to shoulder blade must be gently rounded;
2) tip of shoulder rounded;
3) elbow rounded:
4) wrist rounded
5-7) first, second, and third phalange joints of the hand and fingers all rounded for unimpeded energy flow. No stiff or angular joints.

4) **The Eight Directions and Eight Basic movements** of the Taiji Quan Solo Form:
Ward Off
Rollback
Press
Push
Pull
Split
Elbow Strike
Shoulder Strike
Their relations to the Eight Trigrams.

5) **The "Nine Zigzag Paths,"** through which the energy is mobilized:
1-3)   From Bubbling Well points (first point of Kidney Meridian on sole of the foot) through the ankles, knees, and hip joints;

4-6) then through the lower tip of the spine, mid back, and Jade Pillow at the base of the neck;

7-9)   then through the shoulders, elbows, and wrists.

Only when all of these paths are fully opened can true technique be expressed from the fingers or the palms. As the "Taiji Quan Classic" says, "Form is expressed in the fingers."

After going through all of these "Numbers" the student may well feel it's time to practice "Forgetting!" Yet once examined and thought about, these images will occur to the mind before and during practice and will help correct deficiencies in posture or *qi* flow. They are also in a loose order of progression from the more basic to the more subtle. Once the student has achieved unbroken threading of intrinsic energy through the "pearl with nine winding paths," she or he can dispense with the numbers and return to the One.

Chapter 7

Some Benefits of Practicing Taiji Quan

This is another excerpt from Sung's book, a concise yet very complete treatment of health and other benefits accruing from concerted practice of T'ai Chi Ch'uan over a period of time. I have selected the best points from Sung's chapter and added considerable material of my own.

Some Benefits of Practicing Taiji Quan

Strictly speaking, when practicing Taiji Quan, one should forget all about benefit and loss, advantage, or disadvantage, and just let Nature take its course. If one does the Forms of Taiji Quan daily over a period of years in accordance with the principles of the *Taiji Quan Classics* and has good nutrition in harmony with the forces of Heaven and Earth, all "benefits" will take care of themselves. Nonetheless, as an expedient of beginners, some positive points of the practice are considered below:

1)   Preserving good health.

In China, from olden times, hygienic exercises like Taiji Quan have been specifically recommended by traditional physicians as being helpful in the cure of a multitude of ailments (see below). In industrialized societies, where "brain power" seems to be in such demand and so-called conveniences relieve much of the necessity to engage in strenuous manual labor that earlier generations found necessary merely to survive, Taiji Quan practice can provide the physical exercise so necessary to healthful living.

Those who do engage in strenuous labor will find that Taiji Quan, by distributing blood freely throughout the body, will relieve fatigue caused by repeated overworking of certain isolated muscle groups. (Very few types of work involve balanced activities for all parts of the body simultaneously, combined with mind-intent and deep respiration). Furthermore, focusing the energies of mind / body away from the brain and toward the *dan tian* has always been considered a fundamental requisite of good health in China and Japan. (See the fascinating essay *Yasen Kanna* by the great Zen Master Hakuin). So it is essential to rest the overworked brain for some time every day, allowing thought to be cleared away and energy to flow back to the vital center.

Many Chinese books on Taiji Quan attribute some or all of the following health benefits to consistent practice of Taiji over a period of time:

Blood circulation and glandular activity are improved; muscles and joints are strengthened; the bio-electrical circulation of *qi* is harmonized throughout the meridians and organs. The *wei qi* (external protective *qi*) of the skin is strengthened, so that the skin is soft and glows with health. The nervous system is toned and the internal organs strengthened.

All of these benefits accrue to the practitioner without ever straining the breath or the heart.

Taiji Quan also is renowned for "cultivating temperament," as Master T.T. Liang repeated so often. In fact, he claimed his most profound secret was his ability to "change my students' temperament."

Yearning Chen in his grand compendium on Taiji Quan (*Taiji Quan, Dao, Jian, Gan, San-Shou He Bian, 1943*), describes in typical Chinese fashion the conditions of the body after long practice of the art:

"Your cheeks will glow with a healthy red color; your temples will feel full; your ears will be rosy and your hearing acute. Your eyes will shine with spirit. Your voice will be loud and carry far; your breathing will be steady and even, with no panting.
Your teeth and gums will be strong. Your shoulders will be powerful. Your abdomen will be full and resilient, like the covering on a drum...your footsteps will be light. Your muscles will be as soft as cotton before the intrinsic energy (jin) has become activated; but they will become taut when the intrinsic energy is active. Your skin will be smooth and rosy, and acutely sensitive. "

[Translation by the Author]

The slow motions of Taiji Quan and the movement of the diaphragm traveling up and down massage the internal organs, creating increased blood flow, and stimulating the production of glandular and gastric secretions. Thus, the body's chemical balances are maintained in harmony and the assimilative and excretory functions are facilitated. For further discussion of Taiji Quan and its relation to physical health, see Chapter One, "Some Reflections on the Art of Supreme Ultimate Boxing."

2) **Increasing Physical Potential.**

As one's health increases, one will notice that various physical and mental potentials increase as well. One can work longer without fatigue; one's resistance to heat and cold develops as does one's overall resistance to disease. Likewise, the mind becomes clearer and more alert. Reflexes improve as the transmission of nerve impulses becomes speedier and smoother. The respiration becomes long and deep, enabling one to take long walks or climb hills without becoming short of breath. Many are the stories of ancient Taiji Quan masters who could walk 30-40 miles per day up and down steep mountain paths. As anyone who has practiced Taiji Quan for some time knows, its effects on the legs are considerable; the legs become much stronger, more enduring, supple and flexible. The spine also becomes more resilient and elastic. For many people Taiji Quan has been a specific remedy for spinal problems.

3) **Cultivating Mind and Spirit.**

(In the flowing three sections I follow J.J. Sung's *A Study of T'ai Chi Chuan* rather closely, with a free translation.)

Mind and spirit are the controlling factors in one's life and the basis of happiness or unhappiness. In the present condition of society, much emphasis is given to the study of skills and techniques and the cultivation of mind and spirit are sorely neglected.[How true this is in today's world and educational system!]

Indeed, one might say that the majority of people, to use the old Chinese phrase, "have minds like monkeys (i.e., constantly agitated) and desires running madly like wild horses." Thus, they suffer from all sorts of nervous ailments. The torrent of thoughts, once loosed, is difficult to halt, and the vital energies, squandered in the pursuit of externals, are difficult to re-collect and concentrate.

The principles of Taiji Quan, such as "forget self, follow the other" (i.e., respond selflessly and spontaneously to events), "Keep heart-mind empty like a hollow valley," "Stand erect and centered," "Sink *qi* to the *dan tian*," all indicate ways to concentrate the mind and spirit so that amidst the situations of daily life one does not scatter and disperse one's spirit and vital energies. As the ancients said, this is the starting point of "rectifying one's heart and making one's thoughts sincere."

The more perfect your Taiji Quan, the more deeply it can remain hidden without being made obvious on the outside. In carrying on this cultivation while practicing Taiji Quan, externally let each movement be smooth and harmonious; internally, let your mind and emotions be happy and peaceful. This is the fundamental principle of relaxing the body and calming the mind and spirit. The statement in the "Mental Elucidation of the Thirteen Forms"—"Internally strengthen the spirit of vitality; externally appear peaceful and quiet"—has the same meaning as the above.

In the beginning you must quiet the mind and concentrate the spirit inwardly; later you can strengthen the spirit of vitality. It is most important that all extraneous thoughts be let go; only in this way can your mind and emotions become quiet and the spirit of vitality be directed inward. The lower *dan tian* is the place where mind and spirit can be concentrated. After you have practiced Taiji Quan for a long period of time and have made its principles habitual, you can steady your mind and feelings, increase wisdom, and strengthen physical vitality, to become like pure gold or precious jade.

4) Retarding Old Age and Making Spring Eternal.

The art of Taiji Quan is patterned according to Yin and Yang and is based on the principles of the *I Ching*, continuing the tradition of cultivating the Way handed down from the Yellow Emperor and Lao Tze. The Body of Taiji Quan [the inner qualities of your body, as developed from long practice of Taiji Quan] is generated by nourishing the *qi* and vitalizing the blood. The Function of Taiji Quan [being able to utilize Taiji Quan Applications in self-defense] consists of being light and relaxed, able to neutralize any opposing force. Internally it benefits the five Tsang (solid organs); externally it strengthens the five Fu (hollow organs). Therefore it has the double effect of cultivating Nature and Life and eliminating illness to lengthen one's lifespan. Hence the note appended to Zhang San Feng's "Taiji Quan Classic" states, "May brave men everywhere prolong their years and enhance longevity, and not use the art merely as a means to martial skill."

[The phraseology here, "brave men," referred to a time when the martial aspects of the art were paramount, or at least were regarded as such by certain people. Thus the Taiji Quan patriarch's warning. For our purposes, we should amend it to include men and women everywhere, for women can profit by studying this art and in many cases can absorb its essence more quickly than men can].

The practice of Taiji Quan not only concentrates on the external movements of the body, but places even more emphasis upon the internal cultivation of spirit and development of *qi*. The statement from the "Mental Elucidation of the Thirteen Forms," "First in the mind, then in the body," and from the "Song of the Substance and Function of the Thirteen Forms," "The mind-intent and *qi* are the master and the bones and flesh are (like) the assistants" both clearly indicate that cultivation of mind and spirit must be given top priority in Taiji Quan. The movements of the body serve to strengthen muscles, joints, sinews, etc., but only by developing the *qi* and cultivating the spirit can one nourish one's spirit of vitality. If the body and mind reach the peak of health, this is surely the beginning of retarding old age and making spring eternal.

[There is a classic phrase in Chinese martial arts: "*Lian quan, bu lian gung, dao lao, yi zhi kung.*"
"If you practice only the external Forms and do not develop internal cultivation, in the end you will have nothing."]

Mental disturbances and unrestrained emotions are the source of all illnesses. In practicing Taiji Quan one must first concentrate the spirit and gather the *qi* so that the brain and mind become peaceful and tranquil. After practicing in this way over a long period of time, one will feel that one's mind is empty and free of cares. No confused thought will arise to disturb one and one will remain serene even in adverse external circumstances. Indeed, it is summed up perfectly in the Heavenly Teacher's instruction to the Yellow Emperor (found in the *Yellow Emperor's Classic of Internal Medicine*, Chapter One: "If you are tranquilly content and mind is empty, the true *qi* will accompany you always; if your original vital spirit is preserved within, from where might illness come?"

The Heavenly Teacher further said, "Those who know Tao pattern themselves according to Yin and Yang and live in harmony with the motions of heaven and earth; they carefully regulate eating and drinking; they arise and retire at the appropriate hour; they do not carelessly overtax their energies; thus their external form and internal spirit can be fully nurtured and they can fulfill their allotted span of years." The very highest principle of Taiji Quan practice is contained in four of the above phrases:

"Tranquilly content, mind empty,"
"The true *qi* will accompany you always,"
"They do not carelessly overtax their energies,"
"External form and internal spirit are fully nurtured."

[Author's translations of the passages above]

If you follow these principles, your internal organs will be strong and your spirit clear, old age will be late in coming and Spring will seem everlasting.

5) Avoiding Accidents.

In studying Taiji Quan, training of the way of stepping is most important. After you have practiced for some time, your step will be smooth, even, and firmly rooted; your center of gravity will be secure. In daily life you will find that you walk just as you do in Taiji Quan, letting one foot firmly support the body while the other gently accommodates itself to the ground or floor before it takes the full weight of the body. Your degree of sensitivity to the ever-changing balances of walking and stepping will be increased so that you can even stroll on rugged mountain paths at night without fear of stumbling. Because Taiji Quan trains the mind as well as the body you can gradually cultivate rapid reflexes and responses.

Your body develops a habitual state of nimble alertness. If you unexpectedly encounter an attack or other sudden danger, you can avoid or neutralize it (literally, "avoid the solid, accept the light"), thereby averting disaster. One who has practiced Taiji Quan correctly for many years will have bones that are very strong and solid, yet possess the resiliency of an infant's. If you become involved in an accident, chances are that the injury will be only superficial and will not touch the bones; your recovery will be rapid. Taiji Quan will gradually aid you to rediscover your body's natural potential for self-preservation; if you practice diligently for a long time, you will gradually discover these abilities.

Perhaps this principle is stated most profoundly by the great Aikido master Koichi Tohei in his book, *Aikido, the Arts of Self-Defense* and in a short biographical story describing his time in China as a Japanese military officer.

The story of his military sojourn in China in the late 1930's describes how Tohei had previously studied Judo and Zen for many years. He assumed that his lengthy training in these disciplines would make him impervious to fear.

Yet when he began to cross a river and Chinese snipers opened fire from the opposite side, he experienced gut-wrenching terror. After getting back to the riverbank, he was not only frightened, but even more, he was angry at himself. Of what use, he thought, were all his years of Judo and Zen training, if in a moment of danger, he was reduced to abject fear.

He spent much of the ensuing night meditating on this problem, which became his personal *koan*. By the next morning he had his answer.

When he stepped into the river again and the Chinese snipers opened fire, Tohei simply relaxed completely, and gave his fate totally over to Nature herself, trusting the Universe to keep him from harm. Amazingly, though the soldiers on the other side continued shooting at him, and he noticed the little splashes of bullets landing all around him, he was never scathed.

Over the next few days, he repeatedly bathed in the river, with bullets flying around him each time, but he remained unharmed.

At last, he had proof of his *ai-ki* (harmony with Qi).

Years later, when he wrote *Aikido, the Arts of Self-Defense,* Tohei urged serious students in the art of Aikido (the "Way of Harmony with Qi") to trust fully in Nature for their protection, and to <u>make themselves worthy</u> of this protection from Nature.

He taught that the deepest level of "self-defense" was to be totally at one with the "will of God." The only "enemy" one should fear was to be separated from the will of God, or the Mind of Nature.

The ultimate goal of training was to create a mind of mercy and generosity, that could love even the smallest tree or blade of grass. Only then would the student become a person whom "Nature was pleased to let live."

I feel this is very much the goal of Taiji study as well.

6) Neutralizing Attacks.

[A great deal of information about practical Taiji Quan Application is described in *T'ai Chi Ch'uan for Health and Self Defense* by T.T.Liang. Other excellent references are:

T'ai Chi Ch'uan, Lessons with Master T.T. Liang by my Taiji Brother Sifu Ray Hayward. This book contains many "Secrets" of Taiji Quan Application unavailable in any other book. You can find this book at www.tctaichi.com.

Also see Scott Rodell's *Taiji Notebook for Martial Artists*.]

One should bear in mind that the purposes of Taiji practice were originally therapeutic in nature and that self-defense ability is a by-product, not a principal purpose of practice. The "body" in this case refers to the "Taiji Body", firmly rooted, flexible at the waist, sensitive throughout with unimpeded circulation of vital energy and inner strength to all parts. This inner development requires years of practice, and it is best to let it take its own course. If one observes the principles of the *Taiji Quan Classics*, everything will mature in its own time.

The "function" of Taiji consists first of being able to neutralize opposing forces. Often if a neutralization movement is applied at precisely the right moment, an opponent will fall down solely as a result of his / her own uncontrolled force. Being able to apply Taiji in this way is the highest skill (absolute non-resistance). Next there is the art of counter-attacking, using the correct line, center of gravity, etc., all of which is detailed in the books by T.T. Liang and Ray Hayward. The very best "self-defense," of course, is not to be there when violence is about to occur. Real Taiji function is to be sensitive enough to a situation so that one perceives a potentially dangerous set of circumstances before they fully materialize and can leave the scene in time (see #5 above—being always protected by Nature).

There is a wonderful story of a dialogue between Carlos Castaneda and Don Juan from Carlos Castaneda, *A Separate Reality, Further Conversations with Don Juan,* which illustrates this perfectly.

Don Juan is describing the "warrior's strategy" to Castaneda. Ever the skeptic, Castaneda brings up the imaginary scenario of someone waiting in ambush for Don Juan with a powerful rifle and telescopic sight, with which he could spot him from 400 yards away.

He says that in such a situation all of Don Juan's "warrior's strategy" would be to no avail. Don Juan just starts laughing hysterically. The annoyed Castaneda presses for an answer about how the "strategy" could possibly be of any use.

Don Juan ends the conversation by simply saying that if someone were waiting in ambush for him with a high-powered rifle, he simply would not show up at that time and place.

Perhaps the most important thing is to apply Lao Tze's way in daily life, be simple, unassuming, unpretentious, always guarding the "Three Treasures", frugality, compassion, and refusal to be foremost, so that chances of attracting violence are minimal.

All of the above still does not come close to describing the benefits of doing Taiji every day. There are the aesthetic factors and the simple joy of moving in harmony with the Cosmos each morning and evening. The best thing to do is forget all the above, play out the movements each day, and when the practice has gripped you so you are deeply involved and cannot get out, use these papers as kindling for a cozy fire on a chill winter's evening.

Chapter 8

The *Taiji Quan Classics*

The Taiji Quan *Classics* are the wellspring of correct principles for the art. Said to have been written by the founder Zhang San Feng and his student Wang Zong Yue, their precise historicity is still debated by martial arts scholars. Nonetheless, their importance and relevance for practice cannot be overemphasized. Each line of the *Classics* should be studied, pondered, and incorporated into one's practice in a systematic way. There are also several audiotapes available from www.totaltaichi.com, which offer a detailed, line-by-line 4 ½ hour commentary on the *Classics*, drawn from a live seminar.

Also, T.T. Liang's book, *T'ai Chi Ch'uan for Health and Self Defense* contains a very detailed and practical commentary on the *Taiji Quan Classics*, as does the book *T'ai Chi Classics* by Waysun Liao.

Understanding the principles set down by the Masters of old will really make your practice come alive and will vault your practice to a far higher level. Amazingly, The *Taiji Quan Classics* can be applied to Taiji Solo Form, self-defense, meditation, and Life—utilizing the very same principles in ever-expanding realms of efficacy

The First Classic

The *Taiji Quan Classic*:
Traditionally ascribed to Zhang San Feng

In every movement the entire body must be light and spirited [with a profound connection to surrounding energies of nature and people] and all its parts connected like a string of pearls. The *qi* should be activated (like the beating of a large drum) and the spirit should be refined internally (in calm contemplation). Let there be no excess or falling short, no projection or hollow, no severance or splice. [*Qi* must flow evenly to every part of the body.] The energy is rooted in the feet, springs up through the legs, is controlled by the waist, and is formed [expressed] in the fingers. From the feet to the legs to the waist, all must act as one integrated whole, so that in advancing and retreating one can attain the proper preconditions [body positioning and timing] and the position of strength [relative to an opponent]. If one does not attain the proper preconditions and position of strength, the body will be scattered and in disorder. The cause of this defect must be sought in the waist and legs. [Whenever you feel tense, unbalanced, or clumsy in your Solo Form, check your foot position and alignment with ankles, knees, and hips.] Above or below, forward or back, left or right, the principle is the same: all depends on the mind-intent, not only the external factors [physical exertion in the Form]. If there is above, there must be below; if there is forward, there must be backward; if there is left, there must be right. If one's intention is to go upward, one maintains a downward intent; if one is about to pluck something up and adds a downward energy (to loosen the root), the root can be easily broken and it can be quickly removed. The solid and empty aspects must be clearly differentiated. Each part of the body has its own solid and empty aspects, and the body considered as a whole is either solid or empty. The entire body is smoothly linked from joint to joint; do not allow the slightest discontinuity.

Taiji Quan is also called "Thirteen Form Long Boxing" because its continuous movements flow on unceasingly like a great river or the sea itself. The Thirteen Forms refer to the Eight Trigrams and the

Five States of Change. Ward Off, Rollback, Press, Push, Pull, Split, Elbow Strike, and Shoulder Strike correspond to the Trigrams Jian, Kun, Kan, Li, Xun, Zhen, Tui, Gen. Advance, Retreat, Look Right, Gaze Left, and Central Equilibrium correspond to the Five Elemental Stages of Fire, Water, Metal, Wood, and Earth. All together, they comprise the Thirteen Forms.

Patriarch Zhang San Feng of Wu Dang mountain said, "Let heroes everywhere (use this art) to prolong their years and enhance longevity, not merely as a means to martial skill."

The Second Classic

The Treatise on Taiji Quan traditionally attributed to Wang Zong Yue, Ming Dynasty

Taiji (the Supreme Ultimate principle) is evolved from Wu Ji (Creative Emptiness-absolute non-differentiation). It is the spring of movement and tranquility and the mother of Yin and Yang. In movement it differentiates (i.e. separates into Yin- Yang); in tranquility it fuses into one (i.e. no movement—pure quiescence).

Do not exceed and do not fall short. Follow the other's move by bending [neutralizing in a circular motion]; extend in a straight line [when countering]. When the other employs a strong force and I yield, this is called "moving away" (putting myself out of reach). When I adhere to the other's retreat so that he cannot escape, this is called "sticking." When a movement comes quickly, I respond quickly; when a movement comes slowly, I can respond in a leisurely manner. Although the changing situations may number ten thousand, the principle remains the same.

As one's practice ripens, one will gradually come to understand intrinsic energy. When one has understood intrinsic energy, one will eventually attain spiritual illumination. But without long and arduous practice, one cannot hope to reach ultimate understanding.

The top of the head is held perfectly erect; *qi* sinks to the *dan tian*. Neither lean nor incline. Suddenly conceal, suddenly manifest. When a force is applied to my left side, my left immediately empties; when a force is applied to my right side, my right seems to disappear. When one looks upward (at a master) he seems to become loftier and loftier; when one looks down at him, he seems to sink deeper and deeper. When one advances toward him, the distance becomes longer and longer; when one (attempts to) retreat, the distance becomes exasperatingly short. A feather cannot be added (without your feeling its weight); a fly cannot alight (without effecting a change in balance). The other does not know me, I alone know him. When a hero is without match, it is because he has mastered all of these principles.

In the martial arts there are many other schools. Although their techniques may differ, they are similar in that the strong overcome the weak and the slow must yield to the quick. But the strong defeating the weak and the slow yielding to the quick is the result in innate physical endowments and has nothing to do with study and technique. When "a momentum of one thousand pounds can be deflected with a trigger force of four ounces" it is clearly not strength alone that wins. When an old man (of seventy or eighty years) can withstand the attacks of a host of young men, how can it be due to his speed?

Stand like a poised scale; move like a cartwheel. If your weight is sunk on one side, your movements can be fluid; if you are "double weighted", you will be stagnant (i.e., unable to adapt readily and quickly to circumstances). One often encounters those who, even after years of practice, cannot put their art to practical use and are subdued by others. This is because they have not understood the fault of double weighting. To avoid this defect, one must know sticking and withdrawing, Yin and Yang. To stick is also to withdraw; to withdraw is to stick. Yin does not leave Yang; Yang does not leave Yin. Yin and Yang complement each other. To understand this is to understand intrinsic energy.

After one has understood intrinsic energy, the more one practices, the more refined and perfect (his techniques will become), and if one examines carefully and comprehends in silence, the day will come when one can fulfill one's every wish. The fundamental point is to forget oneself and follow the other. But many mistake this to mean abandon the near to seek the far (i.e. jeopardizing one's own center to attack an opponent's center). This is called making a mistake of inches and missing the goal by a thousand miles. Therefore the student should pay careful attention (and discriminate wisely).

Note: Double weighting can mean:
  1. Keeping one's weight spread evenly on both feet in a static posture;
  2. Using force (weight) to resist force, rather than being "light" (neutralizing) when a force comes to one's body.

The Third Classic

Explication of the Use of the Mind in Practicing the Thirteen Forms, attributed to Wang Zong Yue.

Let the mind mobilize the *qi* so that it can sink deeply and be gathered into the bones. Let the *qi* move the body, so that it may follow freely and heed every dictate of the mind. If your vital spirit can be raised, there will be no defects of slowness or clumsiness; this is called "suspending the top of the head (as if) from a string." The mind-intent and *qi* should interchange in a spirited way so as to develop a rounded and lively tendency; this is called "interplay of solid and empty." In issuing energy one must sink deeply, relax completely, and concentrate in one direction. While standing, the body should be centered, upright, tranquil, and at ease, able to sustain an attack from any direction. Mobilize the *qi* as though threading a pearl with nine zigzag paths; there is no crevice that it does not penetrate. Move the intrinsic energy like steel refined a hundred times over; there is no hard object that cannot be destroyed.

One's appearance is like a hawk about to seize a rabbit; one's spiritual concentration is like a cat stalking a mouse. While tranquil, be like a mountain peak; while moving be like the current of a great river. Store up intrinsic energy like drawing a bow; release energy like shooting an arrow. Within the curved seek the straight; store intrinsic energy before issuing it. Strength is exerted from the spine; steps follow body changes. To withdraw is also to attack; to attack is to withdraw. The energy may be broken off, but is immediately rejoined. In going forward or returning, one uses "folding" technique; while advancing or retreating one must have smooth changes (of body and stance). From developing the utmost pliability and suppleness, one will later arrive at the utmost power and firmness. If one can breathe correctly, one can become spirited and lively. The *qi* must be cultivated correctly to avoid ill effects; the intrinsic energy must be stored up by bending (the limbs), so there is always some to spare. The mind is like the commander; the *qi* is the flag; the waist is the banner. At first let your movements be open and expanded; later make them small and compact, so they can become perfectly refined and subtle. It is said, "If the opponent does not move, I do not move; at the opponent's slightest stir, I move first." The appearance is relaxed, but one is not slack; one is capable of great expansion, but has not yet expanded; though the intrinsic energy may be broken off, the mind-intent remains.

First in the mind, then in the body; if the abdomen is completely relaxed, the *qi* can gather and enter the bones. The spirit is at ease and the body tranquil, keep this always in mind. Remember, when one part moves, all parts must move; when one part is still, all parts are still. When you push and pull, advance and retreat, the *qi* adheres to the back and is gathered into the spine. Internally, fortify your vital spirit; externally, appear peaceful and quiet. Step like a cat walking; move the intrinsic energy as though you are drawing silk threads from a cocoon. Throughout the entire body the mind-intent should be concentrated on the vital spirit, not on the breath. If one dwells too much on the breath, one will be clumsy; overuse of (external) breath will not bring true strength. By not overusing the breath, one can develop unalloyed firmness. The *qi* is like a wheel; the waist is like the axle.

This *Classic* is usually attributed to Wang Zong Yue, a disciple of Zhang San Feng. Stories have it that Wang visited the Chen Family Village and was the first to teach them the principles of Taiji boxing.

The Fourth Classic

Song of the Substance and Function of the Thirteen Forms

The thirteen basic Forms must never be regarded lightly.
The original source of their meaning is in the waist.
In changing from solid to empty and back again, one must pay close attention;
Then *qi* will circulate throughout the entire body without the slightest constraint.

Though one moves to respond to forceful action, one maintains a tranquil attitude.
Manifest your own marvelous techniques only in accordance with the opponent's changing actions.
Pay special attention to your every Form and examine its hidden meaning.
Then you can acquire this art without exerting excessive effort.

Constantly pay attention to your waist.
When your abdomen is completely relaxed, the *qi* will suddenly awaken (and circulate without hindrance).
When the lowest vertebrae are centered and upright, the vital spirit reaches the top of the head.
When the top of the head is held as if suspended from above, your whole body feels light and nimble.

Examine and investigate carefully and thoroughly;
Whether bending, stretching, opening, or closing, follow the natural way.
To enter the gate and be guided onto the proper path, one requires verbal instruction (from a competent master).
If you practice assiduously and study with care, your skill will take care of itself.

If one asks about the correct standard of substance and function, (the answer is that) the mind and *qi* are the Master and the flesh and bones follow.

Thoroughly examine what the ultimate purpose is—
The enhancement of longevity, rejuvenation, and ageless youth.

This Song contains 140 words [Chinese characters].
Each word is genuine and true and its meaning is very far-reaching.
If you do not seek carefully in the direction indicated above,
your time and effort will be spent in vain and you will have cause to
sigh with regret.

[This translation is very similar to the one in T.T. Liang's book,
which I edited, after poring over the original text numerous times
with Master Liang. I have made a few changes in this version].

Chapter 9

"Facing North..." and "The True Meaning..."

The following two articles contain some of the more arcane Taiji lore. "Facing North..." is another excerpt from J.J. Sung's book, and describes what may have been some of the inner lore of Taiji Quan from earliest times, when it was primarily a Taoist art of self-healing, intended to open up the body to higher powers.

"The True Meaning..." should be read line by line without the commentary at first; then read each line singly with the commentary. This also contains much Taoist lore referring to the tranquil mind-spirit state as the source of subtle energies. It deals with the "Fourth F"—the stage of "Forgetting", and thus represents a much evolved level of practice.

Facing North When Practicing Taiji Quan

When we practice the (Taiji) Solo Form, what direction should we face when beginning the Form? In the book *Chen Family Taiji Quan Described and Illustrated* it is suggested, "The North Star and the Big Dipper are both in the northerly direction; the student should face toward them, reverently receiving heavenly counsel, then the Original *Qi* will be in touch with its true ruler." The author (J.J. Sung), speaking from the viewpoint of the principles of the *I Ching*, holds a very similar opinion. Because the North Star is the star Zi Wei (also called Bei Ji star—The North Pole Star) and it also demarcates the superior position in the stellar line-up, the court astronomers in our country's ancient period determined that the North Pole Star was the most honored among the constellations, symbolizing the Son of Heaven [the Emperor] among human beings. The *Astronomical Annals of the Chin Shu* [Book of Rituals of the Chin Dynasty] say, "The heavens revolve endlessly; the Three Luminaries shine intermittently, but the Pole Star does not move."

Therefore it is said, "It dwells in its place and the multitude of stars honor it." And now, speaking from the viewpoint of European knowledge, the North Pole Star is the axis of the heavens; it is the star Alpha of Ursa Minor. Actually it is a double star—one large, one small (Yin / Yang in combination, symbolizing Taiji). It is situated as the most northerly extension of earth's axis line. Seen with the naked eye, it never moves; all the people in the Northern Hemisphere can see it; its position is constant day or night. However, observed through instruments in an observatory, it is actually 1 degree 10 minutes from the true pole, and each year approaches the true pole by 15 seconds (138 years from now it will reach its closest point), but the naked eye cannot detect this.

[This is translated by the Author directly from Sung's book, published around 1970. More recent astronomical information as to the North Star's position and movement would be somewhat different.]

The North Star's position is closest to the North Pole; it is the center point of the revolution of the entire celestial sphere. It is possibly the only genuine great constant star in the universe. Its so-called small double star is nothing more than its satellite. Its magnetic properties have enveloped the entire universe. The True *Qi* that we wish to cultivate in practicing Taiji Quan naturally cannot be unaffected by the Pole Star's magnetic force. Biologists have already discovered that there is a small body comprising a nerve axis near the optic thalamus below our brains that is able to receive the True *Qi* of the subtle magnetic impulses between heaven and earth, influence a person's thought processes, and so have special relevance for those who are refining their *qi*. This part is called our subliminal mind; it is located behind and below the Xin Hui Point (Governor Vessel 22) on the skull just above our forehead, exactly opposite the star's radiance coming from obliquely upward.

In order to more conveniently receive the stimulation from the North Star and the magnetic force from the earth, we must face directly toward the North before beginning to practice the Taiji Solo Form. After regulating the breath, making inhalation and exhalation even, inhale and direct the breath internally to the *dan tian*. Then, begin to mobilize the True *Qi* from the *dan tian* circulating around the Water Wheel, passing through the points on the Governor Vessel, reaching Kun Lun (GV 20, also called Bai Hui on the crown of the head) and going below it to Xin Hui (GV 22) taking in the True *Qi* of Heaven and Earth. [This is a circuit through points on the Acupuncture "meridians."]

This is the violet-hued *qi* of the Pole Star's magnetic force that then passes through the Conception Vessel, returning and concentrating in the lower *dan tian* to warm and nourish it. After that it pulses out to the four limbs in the Beginning Form until, practicing in continuous flow without a break, one reaches the Concluding Form. One then concentrates the *qi*, returning it to the lower *dan tian*, circulates it once more through the Microcosmic Orbit and passes it through the Xin Hui point to inhale and supplement the True *Qi*.

Thus, only by practicing the Beginning and Concluding Forms facing due North can one directly receive the violet-hued *qi* emanating from the North Star. When we look at this slightly violet fluorescence, it makes us feel especially comfortable and happy. (It is also emanated to earth during daytime, intermixed with sunlight). This is a directly perceptible response that everyone knows. Although violet light appears weak when looked at, it has the power to kill bacteria when used medically, and it can also improve a person's disposition. The above is sufficient to demonstrate that facing the North Star does indeed have great benefits for the health of body and mind.

The seven stars of the Big Dipper are close to the North Pole. Of those seven stars, four are called Kuei—the bowl—and three are Shi—the handle. The stars Shu and Xuan (1st two stars of the bowl) are on a direct line that connects the other stars and leads them to the North, to the very position of the North Star. It is as though the revolving movement of the Dipper is receiving the energy of its axial rotating force from the Pole Star. It symbolizes the movements of arms and hands when we practice Taiji, receiving their motivation from the revolving axial energy of the torso.

The star at the end of the handle of the Big Dipper, named Glittering Light, is obliquely opposite the celestial center, pointing out from afar the direction in which the multitude of stars must revolve. Therefore, the Big Dipper represents the compass of the universe; it is the pivot point of movement and harmonizes with the North Star, pivot point of stillness, controlling the entire heavenly body of the universe. It has the same significance as the effect of the two kinds of movement when we practice Taiji Quan, the original body position and original space position. So, in facing North when we practice Taiji Quan, we can unnoticeably develop sensitivity and wisdom going far beyond the mere prolongation of life.

Kan is in the Interior Direction

Taiji is based on the principles of the *I Ching*; the principles of the *I Ching* are based on the He Tu and Lo Shu. [Ancient Chinese cosmological diagrams describing numerological correlations of the compass directions and Five States of Change]. This is the wellspring of our country's culture [China] and is also the original principle behind the movement and quiescence of all things. In both the He Tu and Lo Shu the number 1 is in the North. Although in each the changes and development of the other numbers is dissimilar, nonetheless the beginning of the sequence must unalterably begin in the North. The meaning contained in this number 1 is very profound: it symbolizes the condition existing before the development of the heavens and all the things in the universe. This is called Taiji.

The *Chapters on Nourishing Life* say, "In seated meditation one should face Kan and have one's back to Li [The Trigrams of Water and Fire, respectively] to be able to acquire the True *Qi* of Heaven's first creation of water, to have vitality like that of the Ten Thousand things reaching the movement of springtime." Taiji Quan's source is in the fundamental principles of Taoist seated meditation; while practicing the Form one must face this direction of the primordial chaos indicated by the number 1 of the Taiji—there can be no doubt.

Surrounding the Taiji Diagram is the Later Heaven arrangement of the Trigrams. The Trigram Kan is situated due North and is precisely in the innermost place (facing the viewer) in the sequence, in accordance with the principle that it is water's nature to sink downward. This is exactly in consonance with the position of the number 1 in the He Tu and Lo Shu. Therefore when the ancients drew diagrams, they always established the North precisely in the inner-most position, and the due southerly direction was in the outer position, with East on the left and West on the right [just the opposite of Western compass arrangements]. This has come from the original principle, traditionally handed down from the He Tu/Lo Shu. So in depicting human figures, one can also accord with this idea of placing them facing north, so that we must face South to enjoy them. (Note that in ancient times offices always faced South and stages for drama always faced North; this follows the same principle).

Taiji is the highest level art handed down from ancient times in our country. For this reason the illustrations and descriptions inserted in this book all use the direction scheme that follows the principle of the Taiji as its standard, so that we do not violate the basic idea of the founders of our Taiji Quan form.

NOTE: *The word "office" above refers to all sorts of government buildings, as well as temples and houses of the wealthy. The traditional Chinese house had its main gate and courtyard facing South.*

The True Meaning of Taiji Quan

The original commentary is in italics within parentheses; my commentary is in brackets.

> Without form without shape
> *(forget your self-hood),*
> [Your entire "Form" has now become absolutely unstructured].

> Entire body thoroughly empty
> *(internal and external fuse into one)*

> Forgetting everything, return to the spontaneous,
> *(follow the mind freely)*
> [Move freely, without specific thought or intent].

> A stone chime hangs from the Western Mountain
> *(The sea is wide, the sky is empty)*
> [You feel as centered and majestic as a huge stone bell hanging in a mountain temple].

> Tiger roars, monkey chatters
> *(refine the Yin Ching)*
> [You may hear sounds of internal energy circulation].

> The spring is clear, water tranquil
> *(mind dies, spirit lives)*
> [Your mind is like a still pool of water].

> Reverse the river, stir up the sea
> *(Yuan qi circulates)*
> [Let fire go down and water flow up (as steam or qi)].

> Fulfill Nature (xing), secure life (ming)
> *(spirit is composed, qi abundant).*
> [Correct practice will allow you the lifespan necessary to fulfill your spiritual destiny].

> Anonymous

[This poems describes the state one experiences during the "Fourth F."]

Chapter 10

Taiji, the Multifaceted Art

This is an article of general interest I wrote for a "New Age" magazine back around 1995. It gives a broad overview of the many aspects of learning and practicing Taiji Quan.

Taiji, a Multifaceted Art to "retard old age and make Spring eternal"

Autumnal dawn comes slowly through the sides of the red lacquered pavilion adorning the hilltop in central China. The pavilion is still shrouded in light morning mist, but upon closer observation, shadowy forms seem to be moving and pulsing with the rhythms of the shifting vapors. We see men and women who seem to embody the very patterns of the swirling mists, playing out the stately ancient exercise-art of Taiji Quan

They alternately appear and are concealed again, as they form such postures as White Crane Spreads Wings, Step Back and Repulse the Monkey, Ride the Tiger, and Sweep the Lotus. If we approach closely enough, we hear the delighted morning song of the showbirds who have been brought to the hilltop in their cages for their own morning "exercise."

Though this scene has been traditional in China for centuries, it is beginning to appear in the United States as more and more people learn this invigorating and profound art of physical exercise, meditation, and self-defense. Taiji Quan (more commonly called "T'ai Chi") had its origins in Sung Dynasty China as part of the Taoist system for health, longevity, and "Immortality." According to early Taoist thought, the physical body was the essential residing place for the souls, and once the body's energy was exhausted, the souls would depart, to eventually resolve themselves back into the Tao again, like the dispersing smoke of an incense stick. The object was to keep the physical body intact and vigorous for as long as possible. Though the majority of later Taoists eschewed the idea of literal physical Immortality, the idea of keeping the body as fit and alive as possible remained a central tenet of Taoist practice. The beneficial side effects were a greatly increased lifespan, superb robust health, positive energy, and the constant enjoyment of Nature's wonders which health and vitality engendered.

Nowadays Taiji is practiced worldwide by millions of people, the vast majority of whom play the Solo Form each day as a most enjoyable and invigorating type of physical exercise and stress release. Advanced practitioners usually begin to absorb more and more of its deep meditative benefits. And a relative minority of players train Taiji Quan seriously as a martial art. Originally, however, these aspects of the art were parts of an unbroken whole, to train body, mind, and spirit to the utmost levels of health, vitality, and serenity.

Many of my students over the years have been confused, even upset, about the defensive aspect of the art. We read in the Taoist classics about Taoists' interest in a peaceful, meditative way of life away from worldly turmoil. Why then practice a highly developed and sophisticated martial art? On one level, the Taoists, many of whom lived in remote mountainous locations, needed a method of self-protection from marauding bandits and wild animals. Development of their full spiritual potential could require decades and to have life cut short prematurely would be tragic.

On a far deeper level, however, training in defensive arts was in itself a very practical method of meditative awareness. As one modern Taiji master told an inquiring beginner, "Oh, Taiji boxing—very good meditation. Your mind not be clear, you be hit right away!" We will see shortly how each level of Taiji practice enhances awareness, alertness, and energy. In terms of healthful physical exercise, Taiji circulates blood and vital energy evenly through the body, without causing strain or an overly elevated heartbeat. At the end of a half hour "round," one feels invigorated and refreshed, not exhausted. There may be a light sweat, but no heavy perspiration.

According to Taoist principles, exercise should nourish the body, not deplete it, and the slow movements of Taiji, all composed of circles, alternately exercise and relax each part of the body in unison. As such, Taiji is an unsurpassed curative practice for young and old alike, and can be adapted to any individual's state of conditioning or health. My own principal teacher, T.T. Liang, was given three months to live by his physicians around age 40 and passed away at the ripe old age of 102! He was alert and joking right up till the end.

My own primary interest in the art of Taiji is in its use as a healing and meditative practice from which we can learn more and more about the Tao and its workings. I have been studying the art since 1966 and find it an ever-richer source of insight on many levels — body dynamics, Chinese medical philosophy, psychology, etc. Teaching Taiji has brought me into contact with players and other teachers across the land, and the Taiji community of brothers and sisters is perhaps the most wonderful (and unexpected) "side effect" of training. My main teacher, Master T.T. Liang, always said , "Taiji friends — are best friends!"

Taiji has only been practiced by the public for the last 90 years; before that it was a closely guarded secret, accessible only to Taoist initiates, people in the very few "Taiji families," and the select groups they taught. Traditionally, it was assumed that before studying Taiji, one would be trained in other meditative and martial arts to form a good and necessary basis for study of the "Supreme Ultimate" art of Taiji, which was regarded as the pinnacle of sophistication and subtlety. It is interesting that in the West, most newcomers to Taiji have no previous background in meditative or martial arts whatsoever. This is now often the case in modern China as well, where many professional people or workers take up the art as a means to maintain health, often practicing as a group before work or during breaks.

In my curriculum at the Total T'ai Chi Academy, beginners first complete introductory training in the Five Animal Frolics, the earliest Chinese exercise system still extant, which is some 1800 years old. Devised by the great physician Hua Tuo of the Three Kingdoms Period (200 A.D), the "Frolics" emulate the movements and spirit of the Crane, Bear, Monkey, Deer, and Tiger. The variations of movement for each animal train specific parts of the body (Crane — lungs; Bear — legs, hips, and kidneys; Monkey — muscles and joints; Deer — sinews; Tiger — gripping and leaping power) and encourage embodying the spiritual power of each animal as well. It is an excellent introduction to Taiji, giving a wide variety of movement and feeling, as well as firm stance work and body alignment. The "Frolics" can be practiced as a superb and enjoyable conditioning and strengthening system in their own right. A complete session of "frolicking" takes about 30-40 minutes and energizes every part of the body without creating fatigue.

After completing the Frolics, students learn "Holding the Moon," a standing meditation which develops a firm root in the legs, a strong lower back, and an even flow of energy throughout the entire body. Though the Taoists practiced sitting meditation forms extensively, they always emphasized balance and variety in training methods. Thus there was tranquil practice (meditation) and moving practice (therapeutic exercise forms or martial arts). Within meditation there was sitting and standing internal cultivation, each balanced according to principles of Yin and Yang.

Once introductory training in Frolics and standing meditation has been completed, students begin learning the Taiji Quan Solo Form. There are numerous Styles of Taiji, the best known of which derive from famous Taiji families, who began teaching the art openly during the last 80-90 years. The Chen, Wu, Yang, and Sun family styles are the most widely recognized of the family systems, and there are also Taoist styles which remain largely unknown. The Style I teach derives from the Yang Style and is a long form, consisting of 108 movements, taking about 30 minutes to complete. The movements themselves can be learned in about one year of daily practice, to the point where they can be done enjoyably and with benefit as a healthful exercise. Much more time is required to learn the "application" and internal feeling of each movement to derive the greatest benefit to circulation of *qi* and intrinsic energy.

Though many people have some familiarity with the Taiji Solo Form, and think of the slow-movement exercise meditation as "Taiji," the Solo Form is only one fundamental training method of the Taiji System. After learning the 108 movement Solo Form, students can begin to learn two-person practices to further develop their sensitivity to other persons' energies and to acquire greater refinement of intrinsic vitality. The two-person exercises range from a simple arm circling with wrists connected to the complex, subtle, and beautiful San Shou, wherein two partners train all the movements learned in the Solo Form and see how they relate to another person's energy, alignment, etc. Though a student may be quite proficient in the Solo Form, it is always very revealing to see whether the principles of balance and centeredness have become truly integrated by testing them in interaction with a partner. In addition to being an invigorating exercise, partner work in Taiji further trains refinement of internal energy, sensitivity, and mental alertness.

After the "empty hand" arts have been mastered, one progresses to weapons. The short walking stick, broadsword (saber), and thin double-edged sword forms can be learned, each with its special "flavor" and beauty and its corresponding two-person drills. Now a student moves with greater speed and power and learns how to maintain Taiji principles of relaxation, centeredness, and alertness in the face of "attacks" with weapons. This requires a high level of calm and mental composure. Each of the weapon forms is specifically designed to strengthen some part of the body, or project energy in a certain way, beyond what is possible in the Solo Form alone. At the pinnacle is practice with the spear, which requires a total coordination of power from the entire body. Those who advance to this level may progress to training with a 12-18 foot long spear. In times gone by, the masters would further refine their spear prowess by training on horseback! After all of the forms and weapons have been learned, one comes down to the real root of Taiji and all Taoist self-healing arts — meditation. Breath control and energy development is practiced, then finally one meditates in utter stillness, communing with Tao in a state of calm and simplicity.

For some students, training in Five Animal Frolics, standing meditation, and the Solo Form fulfills their needs for a healthy exercise and meditation. But I have found that many students become more and more enthused and interested in the art as they begin two-person work and weapons training. The double-edged sword form in particular, is beautiful, and embodies real spiritual feeling. Often similar forms or dances were used by Taoist priests in their ceremonies, to symbolize cutting away delusions and purifying the mind.

The entire Taiji System itself is but one branch of the totality of Taoist training for health and long life. Over many years of research, I have summarized the myriad of Taoist practices into nine self-healing or life-arts, which encompass a total spectrum of healing and living in accord with Tao. These are the widest ranging and most complete "holistic" system I have ever encountered. Meditation, Nutritional Science, Movement (including therapeutic and martial forms), Herbology, Acupuncture, Sexual Practice, Geomancy, Divination, and Bodywork (massage, etc.) form a composite whole; each interrelated with others through a common philosophy and outlook. The first three are of prime importance in one's everyday "cultivation" of Tao, and the others are supplementary, to be used as necessary for special situations or adjustments.

My main focus at the Total T'ai Chi Academy is on the movement aspect of the nine life-arts, since that is perhaps the best overall entry point for most people into the philosophy and practice of the Way. The other arts are taught in seminars throughout the year, sometimes by visiting masters. For me personally, practicing the Taoist life-arts, especially Taiji, has been an endless source of delight and inspiration, and a most practical way to learn Taoist philosophy. Aside from producing great benefits to my own health, Taiji has enabled me to meet many remarkable and wonderful people throughout the country, and to enjoy the steady growth of the Taiji "family" in our land. Zhang San Feng, reputed founder and Patriarch of Taiji, may never have envisioned his art of "Immortality," once a closely guarded sacred secret from the Taoist holy mountains, finding its way by the meandering unpredictability of the Tao into YMCA's and street corner parks in America. I am hoping that someday my own personal dream comes true—to be able to go out into any park in the country and see men and women, old and young, practicing Taiji Solo Form, Sword, and two-person arts in the early morning, moving with the rhythms of Nature in joy and harmony, prolonging their years into unending springtime.

Chapter 11

A Letter to a New Taiji Beginner

Since many new students come to Taiji classes with "no clue" as to what learning the art really involves or entails, I wrote an introductory letter to my students. The letter was written while I was teaching at my studio in the hills of Vermont. It was intended to give new students an overview of the practice and their trajectory of learning, as well as some practical advice to maximize the value of their time and study. At that time, my school was known as the Deer Mountain Taiji Health Academy.

September, 1996
Deer Mountain Studio

Dear Taiji Friend,

Welcome as a newcomer to the Deer Mountain Taiji Health Academy! If it were possible, I would like to have an hour or so with you alone to tell you in person what our training in Taiji and the Tao of Health is all about, but since my teaching and seminar schedule is so busy right now, I take this expedient of a written letter to fill you in on the Deer Mountain story, and what you can look forward to in your training here.

What our Name Means

Deer Mountain is my home studio in a solitary corner of southern Vermont, a place conducive to practicing the Tao. There are numerous deer in the surrounding woods, as well as owls, bear, and coyote. The air is fresh and the waters clear. I teach a few of my local students in my home studio, as well as my "Old Timers," who have become part of my Taiji family and are thus welcome in my home. That is the physical place. But Deer Mountain is also a state of mind. The Deer, symbolic of grace, vigor, and agility reminds us of the goals of Taiji training. And the mountain, an abode of peace and tranquility, reminds us of the firm roots of Taiji, as well as the closeness to clouds and stars, so treasured by Taoists of old.

Clouds, composed of wind and water, are manifestations of *qi*, or the vital forces in Nature, and stars are crystallizations of spiritual power. That is why the ancient Taoists and many Taiji masters favor the mountains as their places for training and self-cultivation.

Since "Deer Mountain" is also a state of mind, however, it exists wherever my students gather for training and in the many places I offer seminars nationwide.

What Taiji Training is all about

Taiji is about tapping into the deepest parts of our self, finding our oneness with Universal Energy and its constant changes. Taiji, in fact, means the endless cycle of wavelike energy flow in all things.

It is about getting our bodies into the best condition possible through carefully attending to posture, bone alignment, correct movement, breathing patterns, diet, and thought processes.

It is about studying an ancient art of longevity and rejuvenation to which many men and women have devoted entire lifetimes of research and practice to pass the art down to future generations.

It is about developing an ideal of gracious and long life "far beyond ordinary stages of retrogression and decay" full of joy, wisdom, and positive energy.

It is about developing an unshakable commitment to daily practice of this rare and marvelous art and an unselfish attitude of helping our fellow students who become our Taiji brothers and sisters.

Levels of Practice and Commitment

There are several levels at which you can practice and grow in the art of Taiji

> **First Level: "Checking it out."** Many people's first exposure to Taiji is seeing some relative, friend, or even stranger practicing the slow, balletic movements of the Solo Form and thinking to themselves: "Hey, I'd like to try that!" What most beginners don't know is that the graceful and effortless appearance of Taiji requires a tremendous amount of power and controlled effort. Some people are fascinated and drawn further into the study; others enjoy a tip of the tongue taste of the art and go on their way.

> **Second Level: Beginner to Middle Timer.** Once you have decided to really practice the art on a daily basis, you

become a student, one step up from mere curiosity. Until you can practice the entire Solo Long Form with a certain degree of smoothness and expertise, you remain a beginner. After you have mastered the Solo Form to a certain degree and the principles of Taiji slowly begin to permeate your life, you evolve into a "Middle Timer."

Third Level: Old Timer. Old Timers have a considerable level of proficiency in the Solo Form, have gone on to some level of expertise in two-person work, and usually are conversant with at least one Taiji weapon. More important than mere mastery of forms, however, is "Old Timer's Mind"—where the philosophy of Taiji starts to shine in a person's life. This is a state of mental "mellowness" and unfailing helpfulness to lower level students.

Fourth Level: Associate Teacher. Associate Teachers remain within the Deer Mountain Fold, teach the Deer Mountain curriculum and remain true to the attitudes and ethics which are part of the Deer Mountain way of life and practice. To be an Associate Teacher, one has to substantially master Forms and have a reasonable proficiency in two-person work. More importantly, an Associate Teacher must have a broad knowledge of Taiji history and tradition, and the philosophies which underlie the tradition. Mere mastery of Forms is NOT enough. Beyond this, an Associate Teacher must have a well-developed teaching style and must constantly seek to perfect and hone their teaching abilities.

Any student at Middle Timer level or above who aspires to be a Teacher should make this known to me and I will guide your training accordingly. It will be more demanding and encompassing than that of the average student.

Guidelines for Class Conduct

In China, any art such as Taiji was taught with a certain informal (as compared with Japanese martial arts), yet very well defined, protocol. Here are a few guidelines which will help your practice. You can also review the chapter on Chinese Etiquette for greater detail.

Attend every class. Real emergencies do arise on occasion and will prevent your attendance, but otherwise, plan on attending every class. Don't let fatigue, cold, heat, or other factors give you an excuse for not coming to class. After all, Taiji is a martial art and as such seeks to develop a spirit of courage and indomitable commitment. And your teacher, who experiences fatigue, cold, heat, just as you do, IS there for every class.

If you must come late to class (rarely, we hope), please enter the studio as quietly as possible. This may seem obvious courtesy, but I am always amazed by Taiji students who loudly walk into a class already in progress. One of the ways I know someone is approaching "Old Timerhood" is that if they are late, they come into a class so unobtrusively that the class is barely aware of their arrival.

Pay full attention in class; don't let your mind wander. The more you concentrate your energy and focus your mind, the more energized and refreshed you will feel during and after the class.

Take every instruction the teacher gives (even to other students) as instruction given to you personally. Even if it does not seem to fit in the moment, it may be very meaningful later on, if you just keep an open attentive mind.

Correct or help other students only if asked to do so by the Teacher.

NEVER stand in back of class talking to other students while class is going on. This is extremely rude to the Teacher and would never be tolerated in a traditional (Chinese) Taiji setting.

If the Teacher is giving prolonged personal instruction to one student at a given time, either pay total attention to that instruction, or go on practicing your own forms. Don't just stand around!

If you decide to discontinue study for any reason, inform the Teacher; please do not just "disappear into the night." In Chinese Taiji tradition, this would be extremely disrespectful; and even in America, notifying your teacher of your departure from study is just common courtesy.

Etiquette toward Masters and Teachers

In China, the Teacher was not considered merely a purveyor of information, but had to EMBODY what was taught. The Teacher was the living example of the art or subject he or she espoused. There was a profound art of etiquette between teachers and students. A detailed article on this fascinating art forms an entire chapter of this book. (Chapter 14) Here are a few brief guidelines:

The True Master is often a paradox to American students. In my experience, the masters who have the greatest proficiency in martial arts are often very humble and quiet—not at all the "macho" image portrayed by the media. This sometimes leads students to adopt an overly casual, or even disrespectful attitude toward them.

In general, anyone who has practiced 30 years or more and whose character has matured may be called a Master, though the more mature masters have often practiced 50 or even 60 years. These people should ALWAYS be addressed as "Master..." even though they will generally say that they are not a master. Calling them "Master" indicates your respect for them and their teaching.

Be supremely respectful of the Master's way and pace of teaching. No real master will ever hold back a student unnecessarily. Any good master will have a rationale behind their teaching style and that rationale may only reveal itself to you over a period of time. I have seen so many instances in which students pester their teachers or masters for more knowledge, or complain about their teaching style. If a teacher's style of instruction genuinely is not right for you, you may best be advised to move on. But first, ask the teacher respectfully about WHY the teaching is proceeding as it is. A good teacher will always respond to this type of polite inquiry and the answer may give you some valuable insights into yourself and the art.

If, at some point, you decide to teach the art you learned from your teacher, always approach the teacher to ask permission first. In China not doing this would be unthinkable, and would almost certainly break the student/teacher bond, perhaps even result in a challenge. In America the teacher-student etiquette is much looser than in China, but asking permission is a sign of respect and courtesy. Your teacher might advise that you are still too immature in the art to teach properly, or might give you invaluable guidance on your teaching. (Note what was said above on Teacher Training). I once had a student who informed me she was going to teach some powerful *qigong* and meditative work which she had learned from me a week before in a one day seminar!

Another student who had taken a four hour seminar on the Five Animal Frolics called me to say she "didn't like" some of the movements I had taught at the Seminar, had made her own changes to the Frolics and was now teaching them.

That made me recall a classic quote from the great Wu Style master Sophia Delza, my very first Taiji Quan teacher. Once when I asked her how and why Styles of Taiji Quan changed, and who was "allowed" to change them, she said, "Paul, there are two ways in which changes to Taiji Quan Forms are made. One is because of profound knowledge and the other is because of profound ignorance."

If you decide to teach Chinese arts of health and *qi* cultivation, always remember:

> *100 days—small accomplishment,*
> *1000 days—middle accomplishment,*
> *10,000 days—great accomplishment.*

In general, you should never teach anything you have not practiced daily for at least three years, and that is an absolutely minimal requirement. And also, never teach anything you don't practice devoutly yourself.

Problems or difficulties in your practice

You may find the first few weeks or months difficult; perhaps you will feel clumsy or uncoordinated, though the element of novelty will also stimulate and excite you. Later, as the process goes deeper, you may experience periods of euphoria or periods where long dormant tensions arise to the surface. Don't worry about or get caught up in any of these fleeting phenomena. Look at practice like the play of waves on the sea. Some days will feel absolutely wonderful, as if you are already a Master. Other days you may feel somewhat uncomfortable or stiff. Learning Taiji is NOT a linear process. Accept the rhythms of ease and occasional difficulty in your daily training as a very deep lesson which will apply to every area of your life. You will unfailingly progress as long as you practice daily and remain centered while observing the process.

Remember that above all, the purpose of training in Taiji or Tao is to enjoy life energy. It is much like learning to play a musical instrument. At first it will feel awkward and probably sound terrible. But with concerted practice, you will soon come to enjoy the beautiful sounds you are making. Don't be discouraged, just practice consistently (and with a sense of exploration and even playfulness) and the rest will take care of itself.

My commitment to you is to give you the best of the knowledge I have developed over the past 31 years, to engender a supportive "Taiji family" for you, and, as time unfolds, to point you to other teachers or areas of study, if that is appropriate for your fullest development.

I am looking forward to training with you and walking the endless path of Eternal Spring, as the Tao unfolds for each of us.

With best wishes for your study,

Paul Gallagher, Academy Director

P.S. Creating your own group of nearby "Taiji Friends" for practicing outside of class will enhance your training beyond belief. After the first few weeks of class, your teacher will help you form some local training groups.

Chapter 12

"Burning Questions" from Taiji Students

It has always been customary during my classes to allocate some time before or after physical practice time to discussion of Taiji philosophy and principles, or a period of questions and answers.

One class seemed so engaged and responsive that I decided to ask for their written questions, so that other groups could benefit from the discussion that ensued. I asked for their most pressing or "burning" questions about their practice.

The following questions and answers come from that class and the discussions that followed.

Frequently Asked Questions from Taiji Students

Many of you have submitted your "burning questions" about Taiji. I am very glad you took the time to do this for two reasons:

1) It gives me insight into what your deepest concerns about your own practice are.

2) By sharing the questions and answers with the entire group, we can all enhance and broaden our understanding and practical training in Taiji.

My original intention was to take one or two questions and answer them after each class. But I was very touched by your sincerity and deep interest in the art, your persistent efforts in training which are visible to me each week as you progress, and the high energy and spirit of the group as a whole.

So I decided to do more than just give a verbal answer after class. In deference to your sincerity and spirit, I have decided to take several days to reflect on each question and to write out my observations on all of them, so you will have a permanent record, which hopefully can help you in your studies.

Let's move right ahead!

Here are the questions and answers, selected in a random order:

WHAT IS THE BEST WAY TO CULTIVATE AND BAL-ANCE THE LIFE FORCE?

There is no single best way to cultivate the life force. It depends on numerous factors—an individual's *qi* at birth, their subsequent development ("after birth *qi*"), age, sex, occupation, spiritual aspiration, stage in life, etc.

In Taoist practice there are no fewer than nine major life-arts, which, as a whole, can balance anyone's vital forces and retain that balance for a lifetime. They are: Meditation, Nutrition, Movement

Therapies (one of the best and highest level is Taiji), use of Herbs, Acupuncture, Feng Shui, Sexual Practice (including practices for pregnancy and post-partum), Divination (as in using the *I Ching),* and Bodywork, which includes Chinese bone setting, as well as *tui na* and massage.

To best cultivate your Life Force, you would evaluate your Original *Qi* (your Original Constitution at birth, determined by your basic physical structure and physiological type) and the present condition of your *qi* by a precise analytical process, taking into account a multitude of factors. Then construct your own individualized program of "cultivation of the Tao" to enhance your longevity and rejuvenation.

[More information on this process of analysis is available in my "Master Key to Perfect Health" audio program available at **www. totaltaichi.com.]**

"The Big Secret..."

However, there is one "great secret" for balancing your life force. *LISTEN TO THAT SILENT, STILL VOICE INSIDE YOUR HEAD—YOU KNOW THE LITTLE "CHATTERBOX" THAT IS CONSTANTLY EVALUATING, CRITICIZING, ETC. WHENEVER A NEGATIVE THOUGHT COMES UP. TRY TO NEUTRALIZE IT IMMEDIATELY, SEEING WHATEVER POSITIVE ASPECTS ARE TO BE FOUND IN THE SITUATION. INSTILL AS MUCH POSITIVE ENERGY IN YOURSELF AS POSSIBLE.*

You can surround yourself with white or golden light each morning or evening, or practice the Taoist "Brain Cleansing" meditation to remove negativity. We are all exposed to tremendous negativity via "news," media, etc. The person of Tao is aware of this, and makes conscious efforts to draw in the Light and positive high-frequency energy each day.

Nothing destroys life force more quickly than negativity, so the Taoist is always alert to restore the positive internal energy as quickly and constantly as possible. The question is—what is the best way to do this? Master T.T. Liang always taught that "changing one's temperament" is perhaps the most essential result of dedicated Taiji study. Yet he never described exactly how to go about "changing temperament."

The idea seemed to be that practicing Taiji Quan long enough, and perhaps studying the principles of Taoism, as espoused in Lao Tze's *Tao Te Ching*, would eventually result in the student's being able to "change temperament."

After I had studied Taiji Quan for many years, a friend introduced me to a remarkably precise and scientific way to "change temperament," to "release" negativity from mind and body, and indeed, to achieve Imperturbability. It is known as the Sedona Method, or the "Release Technique." Take a look at **www.sedona. com** or **www.releasetechnique.com** for complete information about this amazing practice. Don't bother about the "hype" on these websites. (I regret to say there IS some marketing hype). Just look for the essence of the method.

The "Release Technique" was developed by a nuclear engineer, Lester Levinson, in the 1950's. Lester had several advanced academic degrees, and was at the pinnacle of his profession. Having had his second massive heart attack at age 42, Lester Levinson was "sent home to die" by his doctors, who predicted he had at best 3 weeks to live. In total despondency, he decided to least discover WHY all his intellectual brilliance had failed him. "If I'm so smart, why am I about to die at 42 years of age?" he asked himself.

He realized that the answer was ENERGY—and how the negative energy he had accumulated throughout his lifetime had not disappeared, but had been stored in his very cells. Since, as a nuclear scientist, he understood the principles of how Energy worked, he experimented tirelessly with ways to release his accumulated negative energy of a lifetime. The ultimate outcome was that he discovered how to "release" his aggregate of negative energy—and went on to live 42 more years in abundant health and left his body voluntarily when he felt his work on earth was done. His story is amazing in itself and can be read on the websites cited above or in the book *Happiness is Free—and It's Easier than You Think* by Hale Dwoskin and Lester Levinson. I have used this technique successfully for many years and it just keeps getting better and better.

WHAT IS THE ESSENCE OF THE RELATIONSHIP BETWEEN MIND AND *QI*, WHICH IS SO FREQUENTLY MENTIONED IN THE *TAIJI QUAN CLASSICS*? HOW CAN ONE BEST EXPLORE THIS RELATIONSHIP IN TRAINING AND IN LIFE?

An excellent question indeed!

Fundamentally MIND AND *QI* ARE ASPECTS OF THE SAME THING.

Each mind state creates a particular *qi* and each movement of *qi* creates a particular mind state. In Taiji Quan, through the series of movements, we move through varied and balanced mind and energy states from beginning to end.

After a while, you may perceive that everything is just a dance of mind states and *qi* states. That is one of the "goals" of Taiji practice itself.

QI is a particular vibration-state of "mind stuff."

It might be called a type of "bio-electricity." Mind is much broader and has infinite states of vibration. The Buddhist classic *Dhammapada* says "All phenomena are fluctuations of mind-substance" or consciousness. In Taiji we direct our "mind," focus it like a beam (our "intention"), and this beam creates a sympathetic vibration in our energy body, and gives the feeling of moving *qi*. Our "physical" body itself is nothing but an accumulation of denser (lower frequency) energies in one place and time, a bundle of energy states held together by the mysterious force of attraction which is our own concept of self.

The denser and more stuck our *qi* is, the more we feel our "self"; when we feel light and completely relaxed, our sense of "self" begins to blend into the totality of things.

For the best description of this I have ever read see the final chapter of John Blofeld's *Taoist Mysteries and Magic.*

This ultimate profound identity of mind and *qi* can be experienced only after long practice of Taiji Quan and meditation.

SHOULD I WORK FIRST FOR RELAXATION, WHICH CAN SEEM UNGROUNDED? HOW DO I VISUALIZE APPLYING A MOVE WITH AN OPPONENT WITHOUT GETTING STIFF? HOW DO I REMAIN RELAXED WHILE PROJECTING FORCE?

Don't "work" for relaxation. It can't be done! The moment you "work," or "try to relax," you are no longer relaxed! Instead let the tailbone, elbows and knees be heavy ("Three Heavies") and concentrate on the smooth, wavelike ebb and flow of the movements.

In visualizing the application of a movement you can again use the image of a wave. Have you ever gone into the surf and been "uprooted" by a huge wave? That is Taiji! Is the wave stiff? Don't think in relative terms about an "opponent."—your body, his/her body, etc. That will stiffen you. Instead project your energy and movement out to infinity as if the "opponent" is but an illusion.

Imagine your forward movements like waves going out into infinite distance, and your intercepting movements catching your "opponent" deftly and smoothly, drawing him/her into your orbit without the slightest resistance or force. This can be done by mastering each element of "Grasping the Sparrow's Tail..."

HOW MANY CIRCLES ARE THERE IN TAIJI?

The Taiji writings say, stretched out, they would fill the Universe, wrapped up they would fit in the palm of your hand.

Every point of every intercepting movement can be the center of a circle. Conversely, if the circumference of a circle is sufficiently large (infinite), it would appear to be straight. You figure it out!!

PLEASE COMMENT ON THE EBB AND FLOW OF IMAGING (TO MOVE THE *QI*), COMPARED TO JUST OBSERVING THE *QI* AND LEARNING FROM IT.

I think at first, you should use imaging to move the *qi* and begin to learn how to sense its movements. Once the *qi* has started to circulate while you do your form, you can either use the Yang approach: deliberately circulate it through imagery. Or use the Yin approach: just observe the *qi* and see how it responds to your movements, breathing, and mind states. Each is valuable in its own time and way. If you are feeling lethargic and unfocused, you can use the Yang approach; if you feel tense and uptight, use the Yin approach.

WHEN SUSPENDING THE HEAD LIGHTLY AND ALERTLY, I NOTICE A CORRESPONDENCE WITH *MING MEN*. WHAT IS THIS ALL ABOUT?

Just as the lower *dan tian* (energy center below the navel) is a focal point for circulation on the front of the body, the *Ming Men* ("Gate of Life" point on the Governing Vessel opposite the lower *dan tian*) is a focal point on the dorsal surface. Suspending the crown lets the spinal vertebrae and Governing Vessel be stretched out and opened. If your circulation of *qi* is already fairly well established, you may feel circulation in and around *Ming Men*.

"ALL EMANATES FROM THE WAIST." DO YOU CONSIDER THE WAIST TO INCLUDE THE *YAO* (INGUINAL FOLDS) OR THE ENTIRE ABDOMEN?

Generally the waist and "crease" (inguinal folds) move together. However, in some movements of Taiji (e.g. Repulse Monkey) and in other internal arts such as Ba Gua, the waist is sometimes distinct from the crease. The crease forms the solid, relatively stable base, which supports the rotations of the waist.

I OFTEN FEEL TIRED OR CONGESTED AFTER PRACTICING. WHY IS THIS AND HOW CAN I PREVENT IT?

This can arise from a variety of causes. First, you may be straining a bit, in subtle ways. Don't try to move the *qi* too deliberately; instead imagine your body pervaded by a warm steam which moves the limbs effortlessly.

Your channels of energy ("meridians") may be obstructed either mechanically or energetically. It may be good to practice the Eight Brocades for a while to open the channels. Also be sure your diet contains predominantly whole, fresh foods with plenty of *qi*. The more processed and packaged something is, the less natural *qi* it contains. If your diet has an excess of sugars or "*qi*-less" foods, you will become congested and fatigued.

Check with a nutritionist as to whether your mineral balance — specifically calcium and iron is correct.

Sometimes people do feel tired for a few minutes immediately after practicing. In this case, slowly pace around for a bit right after your Solo Form, then sit for a few minutes. Often after a very brief initial period of fatigue, you will feel vastly energized after Taiji.

Perhaps the class is more demanding and lasts longer than your regular personal practice. Be sure to practice daily!

WHAT WORD BEST DESCRIBES OR CAPTURES THE SPIRIT OF TAIJI?

The *Taiji Quan Classics* say, "One's appearance is like a hawk about to seize a rabbit; one's spiritual concentration is like a cat stalking a mouse."

I would call it moving at ease through the Ten Thousand Changes or wandering freely through vast emptiness. (The latter is stage four of the "Four F's." See Chapter 6, "Taiji By The Numbers.")

I HAVE EXPERIENCED MY ARMS SEEMING TO LIFT BY THEMSELVES IN THE BEGINNING FORM AND PLAY LUTE AND I FEEL A BALL OF ENERGY IN THE *DAN TIAN* WHILE DOING SOME OF THE CRANE MOVES. HOW CAN I MAINTAIN, ENHANCE, OR ENLARGE THESE SENSATIONS?

The best way is simply to do each movement with full attention and awareness, with a relaxed spirit. One of my teachers said that feelings such as you describe will first "come around once in a while to knock at the door..." then may disappear for a while. Gradually you will feel a specific energy in every movement of Taiji Quan, but this will take some time.

Still later, the specific feelings of *qi* flow may be supplanted by an overall sensation of warm inner circulation and comfort that is less specific than before. You may find at some point that the feeling of effortless spontaneous movement occurs at various places in the Solo Form. This is excellent, but will usually not be consistent throughout the entire Form (it is always more difficult in the kicks). The main thing is to remain mentally and spiritually at ease during the entire process, watching and gently guiding the energy flow rather than trying to control it (a subtle distinction). Remember the Taoist maxim of *wu wei*, acting freely, never forcing something to go against its natural flow.

DOES THE SELF DISAPPEAR WHEN TAIJI IS DONE CORRECTLY?

What we call the "self" is a collection of tendencies—mental, spiritual, physical. Our internal or physical tensions also give us more sense of "self." When we are profoundly relaxed our sense of ego-self tends to diminish, in favor of our grander Self, which encompasses numerous dimensions. This is one of the major "goals" of Taiji training.

The more correctly Taiji is done, the fewer physical tensions or imbalances will arise to impede the development of the grander Self.

HOW DOES THE TOTAL ASPECT OF TAIJI- MENTAL, PHYSICAL AND SPIRITUAL—MANIFEST ITSELF IN EVERYDAY LIFE AND CREATIVE ENDEAVORS— ART, ETC.? HOW DOES TAIJI PREPARE YOU FOR LIFE AFTER LIFE?

The long-term practice of Taiji results in an attitude—above all, a "change of temperament." This equitable temperament manifests throughout everyday life in ways too numerous to mention,—in work related matters, family relationships, etc.

Also, if we are always feeling healthy and positive, our natural magnetism will affect people around us and they will feel better also, thereby returning good feelings to us. It is an energizing cycle. If we can maintain excellent health for our whole life, not only will that benefit us in so many ways, but we will not be a burden to others and can instead imbue them with more healthy vibrant energy. Two of the people who have most inspired me in this regard are my father, who at age 80 and after 9 heart attacks (and being on the brink of death on several occasions) still lives a positive, adventurous, and happy life. Though his health is surely compromised, his mental attitude is unfailingly positive. He is still working, writing his memoirs and poetry, and traveling widely.

[He passed away peacefully, with a prayer on his lips, at age 81.]

The other inspiring mentor is my principal Taiji Quan teacher Master T.T. Liang, who at age 91 is still healthy, alert, strong, and good-humored. He has often said that his goal is to enjoy the beauties of life right up to the end, and then pass away with a smiling face.

[Master Liang passed away peacefully at age 102. He was very alert, lively and healthy on the great celebrations of his 100th birthday——and blew out all 100 candles on his birthday cake with one puff!!—- amazing!]

I do not have much experience with artwork, but in theory the relaxed, flowing, centered movement of Taiji is directly applicable to the brush and other arts. I think this is a function of relaxation, centeredness, and sensitivity. Many famous Taiji Quan masters, T.T. Liang and Professor Cheng Man Ch'ing as prime examples, were also outstanding calligraphers and painters. They had both mastered the *Wen* (Cultural) and *Wu* (Martial) aspects of life.

If we do Taiji long enough to become completely relaxed inside — physically, emotionally, and spiritually, it will facilitate a smooth "liftoff" when it is our time to leave the physical realm. Otherwise, tensions and the emotional energetic residue of "unfinished business" will tend to block the powerful energies needed to vault into the empyrean. Taiji develops a lot of energy, keeps the channels open for smooth circulation, and de-stresses body and mind so that we can more freely leave the physical world in our energy body when our work on earth is done, to explore further realms for spiritual enlightenment.

WHAT IS THE CONNECTION BETWEEN THE LOWER, MIDDLE, AND UPPER *DAN TIAN*, AS IN "HOLDING THE MOON?"

Each of the *Dan Tians* has its own vibratory speed and way of converting energy.

[*Dan tian*, literally translated as "field of the elixir of life," is an energy center of the body in which *qi* gathers and is transmuted into higher or lower frequencies.]

Lower *Dan Tian* (situated below the navel) is the slowest and most "physical," being concerned with generative and nutritive forces and overall level of physical energy.

Middle *Dan Tian* (in the Solar Plexus area) joins physical with emotional and has a higher vibration.

Upper *Dan Tian* (in the "Third Eye" area) has the most rarified vibration, is the seat of Spirit, and connects us with psychic input or the more subtle realms of existence.

In "Holding the Moon" (a form of standing meditation) we start at the middle, joining some aspects of physical vitality, emotion, and spirit; then conclude by letting the energies find rest in the overall reservoir of original body *qi*.

I AM HAVING SOME DIFFICULTY PRACTICING THE FORM SLOWLY, SOMETIMES IT FEELS LIKE IT'S "DYING." PLEASE COMMENT ON SPEED DURING PRACTICE

The Chinese say the Solo Form "must not be too slow or too fast." The idea is to move like the ongoing flow of a river or stream. Moving too slowly may stagnate the *qi* and necessitates more endurance in the legs and heart. Moving too rapidly may cause body tensions and hurried breathing. The more proficient your practice is, the slower you can go and still retain even flow of *qi*. For beginners it is best to take a middle speed, just so that it feels flowing. The energy must feel comfortable and light. As the *Taiji Quan Classic* says, "The entire body must be light and spirited and all of its parts connected like a string of pearls."

Try to get a smooth, centered, flowing feeling rather than trying too much to move the *qi*. Trying too hard to move the *qi* will result in tension and stagnation. Keep the attention centered on the spirit and the flow rather than on *qi*. "Throughout the entire body the attention should be concentrated on the vital spirit, not on the qi." (Wang Zong Yue's Classic, "Elucidation of the Mind-Intent In Taiji Quan")

WHAT IS THE DIFFERENCE BETWEEN QIGONG AND TAIJI?

Qigong can refer to any one of literally hundreds of different exercises to develop or circulate the *qi*.

There is healing *qigong* to cure or fortify the internal organs; there is martial art *qigong* to enable the practitioner to project huge amounts of concentrated power, or even to withstand fully focused strikes to his/her own body. There is spiritual *qigong* to refine the *qi* to a higher level in preparation for advanced meditative techniques.

In very general terms, *qigong* is more specifically focused than Taiji and often can develop *qi* more quickly and intensely. Usually forms of *qigong* are less complex and subtle and easier to learn than Taiji Quan.

Taiji Quan is a "global" form of *nei gung* (internal energy cultivation). That is, it affects the entire body as one undivided whole. The effects of Taiji Quan are developed gradually and last a long time.

As one master said, "*Qigong* is like getting wet in a rainstorm; Taiji Quan is like getting wet by walking through dense fog."

That is all of the queries I have received to date. For me, taking a number of hours to reflect on and respond to these questions has been rewarding in its own way, compelling me to clarify many experiences which have crystallized in my own practice over the past 30 years [in 1997].

I hope the above is rewarding and useful for you as well and gives you an insight into the incredible depth and magic of Taiji cultivation of the Tao. It is with good reason that it is called the "Supreme Ultimate" exercise because it works simultaneously on so many levels and causes enduring changes in physiology and spirit.

Thank you all for the sincerity of your practice and for the fun and good feeling of working with you on Wednesday nights.

Yours for "Eternal Spring" through Taiji

Paul

Chapter 13

The Taiji System

When most Americans hear the word, "Tai Chi," they immediately think of the slow, balletic movements of the Solo Form, and of an exercise that is for relaxation and alleviation of stress. It would defy belief for most Americans to hear that Taiji Quan is a formidable martial art that was formerly taught to the Chinese Emperor's elite personal bodyguards.

While relatively few modern practitioners (either Chinese or American) delve deeply into its martial aspects, the fact remains that Taiji Quan is a total system of mind-body development. It is extremely sophisticated in its principles and training methods. Although many American students seek Taiji for its benefits as a form of stress release and gentle exercise, it is still very important to seek instruction from a teacher who is acquainted with the martial "Applications" of Taiji. And the teacher should also be versed in at least some aspects of the entire "System." Otherwise, the student will be able to glean only a very small fraction of Taiji Quan's real potential for overall mind and body development.

It is also critical for the Taiji student to become at least familiar with the martial Applications of the Solo Form. Only by imaging and having some awareness of the "Applications," can a student experience a genuine flow of *qi* in the Solo Form.

Many students, coming to practice for the relaxation benefits of Taiji, studiously avoid any practice or even awareness of the martial aspects. This is a big mistake. Always remember Taiji Quan seeks full development of the entire person. If your goal in study is solely for exercise, you need not assiduously practice the Applications for real-time use in combat, but you must at least know how each movement of the Solo Form CAN be used as a martial art. Otherwise your

Solo Form will be an assemblage of pretty movements and will not effectively circulate the internal energy.

Taiji develops the whole person in Yin and Yang aspects. Correct study of the art makes an overly Yin (timid, weak, or retiring) person strong, and an overly Yang (aggressive, belligerent, hyperactive) person more balanced and relaxed. The majority of American students who come to Taiji seem to be on the Yin side, and then most teachers teach them to be even MORE Yin with the constant admonishments to relax, slow down, etc. That is because many American teachers really lack any knowledge of Taiji's Yang side. Remember, the master teacher's job is to create a more perfect balance in the student. The old teaching proverb says, "Where there is Yang, create Yin; where there is Yin create Yang." So just remember that your teacher should be able to teach both aspects of the art as your learning curve progresses.

What Is The Taiji "System?"

Many new students, especially young and athletic ones who have studied with me over the years have asked whether Taiji is "aerobic," whether it builds strength, or whether it is compatible with weight training. These common questions are asked because most beginning students (and most Americans in general) think that "Taiji" is nothing more than the slow Solo Form.

Only when a person understands that the Solo Form is but one part of the Taiji System can they see the real potential of Taiji as an unexcelled method of development for the entire body, as well as mind and spirit.

Though there is certainly no single, exclusive Taiji System even among adherents of a particular Style, I have come to consider the following elements as essential to realizing the fullest potential of Taiji practice, for internal healing and longevity, self defense, and ultimately, spiritual development.

"Empty Hand" Training Includes the Following:

1)   <u>Stage One — Basic Conditioning</u>

The aspiring student can benefit from conditioning exercises for strength, flexibility, and coordination. It never fails to amaze me that a system of exercise which was once the exclusive province of high level martial artists or Taoist priests, who were assumed to have mastered a widely encompassing range of physical skills or martial arts prior to studying Taiji (the "Supreme Ultimate"), is now commonly available to people with no previous physical training whatsoever.

Older beginning students usually need a lot of help with gaining leg strength, flexibility, and coordination, while younger beginners often move stiffly, or use too much muscular power. For both groups, a series of initial exercises proves extremely beneficial. One of the best is the <u>Five Animal Frolics</u>, which provides complete body conditioning, as well as acclimating the beginner to slow movements with relaxed breathing from the *dan tian* (center point of body energy, just below the navel). Another is the famous <u>Eight Brocades</u>, which are excellent internal stretches and teach the rudiments of correct respiration.

2) <u>Stage 2 — Standing Meditation</u>

After basic conditioning exercises comes Standing Meditation, such as "Holding the Moon" or "Embracing the One." Standing is essential to gather *qi*, create a strong <u>root</u> (a firm and unshakeable stance) , and begin to restructure the body frame — the alignments from shoulder to hips, to knees, to ankles upon which the proper use of body mechanics in Taiji (and all internal martial arts) depends. Standing meditation is done with a feeling of calm indomitability; you hold your ground with the dignity and stature of a mountain at rest. There are several standing postures I generally use in teaching, mostly derived from the *I Quan* (Mind-Intent Boxing) system.

3) <u>Stage 3 — Single Leg Standing</u>

When the student has developed strength in the legs, and has learned to calm the mind and breathe correctly through "Holding the Moon," it is time to begin practicing single-leg standing. Using a posture similar to the Yang style "Raise Hands and Step up," the student begins to sense the yin/yang balances in the body — solid and empty in the legs; forward and backward; right and left; and the contrast between the energies of the lead and trailing hand. Once the single leg standing is mastered and can be held for 5 minutes on each side, the student further perfects the sense of balance by walking, from standing on one side to standing on the other. There is forward walking, based on the posture resembling "Raise Hands and Step Up, and a backward walking based on a posture similar to "Play the Lute."

Single leg standing really develops root and endurance, and the walking transitions greatly facilitate a control of solid and empty aspects of weight shifting to create perfect balance while stepping.

4)   **Stage Four—The Four Essential Movements**

Once the groundwork has been completed, students can learn the Four Essential Taiji Quan Movements—"Ward Off, Roll Back, Press, Push," in a repetitive circular format which is done to both sides.

5)   **Stage Five—The Eight Essential Movements**

This is followed by a similar variation with the Eight Taiji Essential Movements, including "Pulldown, Split, Elbow and Shoulder Strikes." Now at last the student is ready to learn "the Solo Form."

6)   **Stage Six—"The Solo Form"**

This what most people associate with the name "Taiji." I generally teach a 60 movement version of modified Yang Style first, then the Classical 108 "Long Form" movement variation.

7)   **Stage Seven—Push Hands**

Following the "Solo Form" comes Push Hands, beginning with the single hand circling, followed by a simple form of circling in which each partner attaches and adheres to the other's elbow and wrist. Then comes Fixed Step Push Hands using the Four Essential Movements, and finally Moving Steps Push Hands.

8) **Stage Eight — Da Lu**

Next comes Da Lu, which begins to teach a greater range of spatial relationships with one's partner, and which emphasizes use of longer range stepping (Roll Back, Pulldown) and short range (Elbow and Shoulder) techniques.

[You can find a DVD on the "Applications" of the Eight Essential Movements at **www.totaltaichi.com.**]

9) **Stage Nine — San Shou — prearranged Attack and Defense**

The last element of empty hand training is the San Shou, or Taiji two-person "Dance," as Master T.T. Liang called it, which includes 156 movements and demonstrates the applications of the Solo Form, as well as ways to neutralize them. Each movement of the San Shou makes explicit the three elements of every Taiji movement: *Hua* (neutralize), *Na* (control), and *Da* (issue energy or attack). After practicing the San Shou, one's Solo Form feels incomparably richer and deeper than ever before. San Shou refines even further the use of timing and correct distance in relation to one's partner, and the joint twisting and locking movements create flexibility and strength in the joints and connective tissues in a way that can never be done through the Solo Form alone.

For those who really intend to master Taiji Quan as a martial art, the San Shou is followed by actual free-style sparring, so that the principles learned in the Solo Form and San Shou can be applied in real-time simulated combat. A very few Taiji Quan masters also teach *pai da* techniques, to make the body impervious to a fully focused strike, if neutralizing the strike should fail.

This completes the "empty-hand" training, that is — training without weapons. In addition, at various times during the previous training, the student can use certain specialized exercises to ensure that s/he is developing the Taiji Quan "body" (*Ti*), as well as "function" (*Yung*).

Specialized Exercises

Practice of various Rooting Exercises is essential to understanding the three major internal aspects of the "Taiji Body" for complete development in the art.

Three Aspects of the "Taiji Body"

1) **Central Equilibrium:**

    This is developed by specific exercises to develop an immovable and powerful stance or "root." The Standing Exercises mentioned above are one of the best methods. This is the most important aspect of training the Taiji Body.

2) **The Yin aspect:**

    Developed by practicing "Willow Bending" exercises, in which a student simply yields to a push from any direction, while maintaining a firm root in the "Bow Stance."

3) **The Yang aspect:**

    Developed by practicing "Push" with a partner who folds elbows across his/her chest and goes with the Push, neither rooting nor neutralizing. These are fully focused "Pushes," in which the person pushed lets the energy propel him/her backwards, while keeping the body in alignment and integrity.

Taiji Classical Weapon Training

This is the second tier of the total Taiji System. Training with Taiji weapons develops the ability to use the body as a concentrated unit and to project energy, while also developing endurance and courage (imagine the old Masters who regularly dueled with live blades!).

1)   <u>The Cane</u>

The Cane, though not originally a Taiji weapon, is a relatively simple instrument that teaches the student to project energy, and understand the difference between arm strength and total body power, Students watching each other perform the Cane set can readily perceive this difference. The Cane also teaches correct usage of the wrist in handling a weapon, a skill that is transferable to study of the Saber and Sword. The Cane Form is done much more rapidly than the Taiji Solo Form, and creates endurance with deep relaxed breathing as well as springy power in the legs.

2)   <u>The Saber</u>

The Saber Form creates suppleness in the waist and power in the legs, develops energy in the wrist and palms, and creates a unified flow of power from legs through the waist and though the wrist into the palm and weapon. The movements of the Saber Form have in them the energy of a fierce tiger, with broad and open chopping and slashing movements, which create a powerful connection between legs, waist, and arms. It is worth remembering that some of the old Masters practiced with sabers weighing many pounds to develop tremendous power in the wrist and torque ability in the waist.

3)   <u>The Double-Edged Sword</u>

The Double Edged Sword Form is the most subtle and beautiful of all Taiji weapon forms. Its energy is that of the dancing Phoenix. The Sword Form develops the flow of *qi* into the fingertips, and projection of spirit to the eyes and tip of the sword. It also develops dexterity and finesse, with subtle movements of the waist and wrist.

The Sword is the most spiritual of the weapons, frequent companion of the Taoist adept, scholar, and high-ranking official of old China. Practice of the Taiji Sword Form leaves one with an unequalled sense of exhilaration and mental peace. The Sword was frequently used in Taoist rituals to summon spirit power, as well as to dispel demons and illusions.

The cane, saber, and sword all develop strength in the tendons of wrist, elbow, and shoulder and affect the smaller muscle groups which are not always exercised in the Taiji Quan Solo Form.

4) **The Long Staff or Spear**

The Spear is the most formidable and demanding of the weapons. Practice of the Spear (or long staff) develops unified power throughout the entire body and trains the legs, waist, shoulders, and arms to issue power in an unbroken wave of synchronization. Starting with an 8 foot spear, one can work up to a 12 foot one, and eventually, perhaps emulate the generals and masters of old, who practiced with an 18 foot spear!

Spear practice develops tremendous unified power and ability to issue energy for a long distance, making the tip of the spear vibrate and the horse tail attached to it swish with a unique sound. Anyone who wonders whether Taiji is "aerobic" should do 100 consecutive thrusts with a 12 foot spear! Use of the spear is the "power training" of the Taiji System.

[For instructional DVD's on the Taiji weapons, see **www. totaltaichi.com**].

Cultivation of Internal Energy and Spirit

Finally, upon completing the physical arts of Taiji, the student learns specialized breathing exercises, based on Taoist techniques to balance fire and water in the body, and create respiration that fully absorbs *qi* from the air and promotes profound tranquility.

The most advanced level of breathing technique merges with meditation, in which the advanced practitioner sits with body, breath, and mind in a state of complete relaxation and attunement with Tao.

Mastery of the complete Taiji System takes an absolute minimum of ten years dedicated study and is a complete and unexcelled system of mind/body/spirit development. There are, however, few students who will follow this path to its rewarding end. Most are content with more modest goals of health and "relaxation." These students are usually taught some introductory exercises, the circular Four Essential Movement set, "Holding the Moon" in its most basic variant, and the 60 movement Taiji Quan Form.

For the relatively few students who learn the entire system, however, the rewards are great indeed and create lifelong health, robust fitness, and serene mental clarity.

Chapter 14

Chinese Etiquette

One of the most important yet least understood aspects of studying Taiji is the art of respecting the teacher. In the China of old and even to a lesser extent today, proper etiquette between student and teacher is essential to creating the environment in which a close bond with the teacher can be established, and learning in depth can take place.

"Learning in depth" because without the extra bond and confidence the teacher feels from a student who practices correct etiquette, the teacher will usually teach only the exoteric aspects of the art. The more profound inner aspects of training will generally be revealed only to those students with whom the teacher feels confident and fully at ease. Proper etiquette on the part of the student is absolutely necessary for this to occur.

Moreover, etiquette is a fascinating art in itself, and its principles will begin to be felt and to enhance many other areas of a student's life outside of the Taiji training studio. It is a most rewarding pursuit and a lifelong fascination to explore and practice.

Here are a few rudiments of Taiji etiquette from a westerner who went through a long and sometimes painful learning curve with very tolerant teachers.

"Filling The Teacup"—the Little-Known Art of Chinese Etiquette

A guide for Chinese martial arts students...

I was a young college student and had decided I wanted to learn Karate from a well-known master in the Boston area in the early sixties. The master, an American recently returned from years of study in Okinawa, was very traditional in his attitude. One could not simply sign up for classes, but had to first be sponsored by another student and then have a personal interview with the teacher himself. So on the appointed day I appeared at the *dojo* in an older building on the south side of Boston and, with a mounting feeling of expectancy, climbed the long flights of stairs. I entered the office area, which was furnished in classical Japanese manner with straw *tatami* mats, a *tokonoma* (ceremonial alcove for flowers and calligraphy), and a low table. My first introduction to Japanese furnishing!

The master was nowhere to be found, so I seated myself on the table, which I took to be a bench, and waited. A few moments later the master appeared and stood at the office door with an expression of shock and amazement on his face. " Please do not sit on the table!" he said in an angry voice. Thus began my education in martial arts and martial arts etiquette. One of the lesser-known aspects of the total art of Taiji Quan is the study of proper etiquette. This encompasses both etiquette relevant to the study of martial arts and the larger scope of Chinese old-style etiquette in general, the art of harmony and respect for one's family and teachers. Although Taiji Quan as a system of martial art and personal health cultivation is based mostly upon Taoist principles, the interrelations of teacher and students are based squarely upon Confucian standards of etiquette. A main tenet of Confucius was that careful attention to one's behavior in the outer world would create a corresponding change in one's inner psychology and attitude. By cultivating awareness and harmony in external relationships, one would develop awareness and harmony within oneself.

"Etiquette" is an Art in Itself

Over the years, I have found this aspect of the art to be fascinating in its own right and though I have acquired some of the rudiments of proper behavior, I still have much to learn. Anyone who has the wonderful opportunity to study Taiji from masters trained in the old school (now an almost extinct group) will soon come to see the importance of this often neglected "secret" of our art. Despite the many modernizations in present-day mainland China, much of the traditional courtesy remains, especially among the older people, and it is particularly important in the old-style martial arts schools which still exist there. To a Chinese of the "old school," education means something quite different than it means to the average westerner.

Here, we seek information, pay our money, get what we want and move on. In a school setting we pay our tuition, study what is required, pass exams or write papers, and move on. In the traditional Chinese attitude, education on whatever level is essentially about how to live, how to be a cultivated human being in the best sense of the term. The teacher, therefore, is not merely a purveyor of information or skills, but must embody the skills he or she teaches, and be a living example of the teaching itself. Entering a school or asking a teacher for instruction is more than a request for information; it is in a sense entering a family.

The Taiji "Family"

There is a vertical and a horizontal dimension. Vertically, there is the lineage of masters and students which goes backward in time to the founder of one's system or school and forward to one's own students and their students. Horizontally, our fellow students are brothers and sisters, whom we care about and treat as members of our extended family. Not only does practice of Taiji create deep spiritual changes in us, but the association with our "family" members creates a spiritual bond uniting everyone in the school. Although few contemporary Chinese Taiji Quan teachers seem to mention this outright, any traditional master one is likely to study with has this family concept in mind, at least subliminally. And invariably, when a student demonstrates knowledge of proper courtesy and respect, it not only creates greater harmony within and between schools, but encourages the master to feel more at ease about giving some of the inner teachings, the real essence of a master's art which has been ripened through decades of practice and self-cultivation.

Two Essential Principles

The following will be a guide to principles of Taiji "courtesy," often illustrated by true to life stories. Many of the stories involve the author and his progress from a totally uncouth "western barbarian" to one familiar with at least the rudiments of "civilized behavior" — from the Chinese viewpoint. There are two fundamental principles underlying the entire spectrum of Chinese etiquette: **modesty** and the creation of *guanxi* (pronounced gwan-shee) or personal relationships based on trust and regard for the other's well-being. Modesty is a quality common to both Confucian and Taoist ways of life. One always praises and compliments the other's abilities, house, children, etc., while diminishing one's own. Quite different from the Western way! This need not become exaggerated or phony, but is more an air of deference to the Master, his or her family, senior students, etc. Again, this can be done very unobtrusively and almost casually. Here is one example. It is very immodest to demonstrate for a master unless requested to do so. When requested, it is very disrespectful <u>not</u> to demonstrate.

Modesty

On one occasion, I went to visit the well-known grandmaster T.T. Liang with a dear colleague of mine and another well-known (and very traditional) master. After the initial greeting and polite conversation, Master Liang asked one of his senior students to demonstrate a sword form, thus expressing his courtesy toward his visitors. After the demonstration was over, my friend went over to the weapon rack on the wall, took down a sword and asked me to assist him in demonstrating a two-person sword set he had just barely learned from the other master. I declined, since I had never even seen the form before, let alone practiced it. My friend became more and more insistent, so finally I acquiesced to avoid creating an embarrassing scene. Our "demonstration" was ludicrous, since my friend had to coach me in every move, teaching me on the spot. All this while the two masters sat looking on! Finally the visiting master yelled, "Stop!!" He rushed over, grabbed the sword out of my hand and attacked my colleague vigorously with movements from the two-person set. End of "demonstration."

When one master pays a courtesy call on another master whom he does not know, there is always some undercurrent of wonder about what the visit really means, what motivations may lie behind it. Chinese are very concerned with what lies behind the surface of things. An old-time master would wonder, "Why is this master visiting me?" In the old days, challenges would frequently arise out of such visits. On this occasion, the students of these masters brought them together in friendship and the meeting was very cordial. Still, I know there was some wonder in the minds of both masters as to what it was really all about.

When Master Liang's student had finished demonstrating, the other master might have asked his student to demonstrate in exchange. Even this might have been a little questionable, since it is unseemly to upstage one's host. When the student demonstrated without invitation, it was very bad form, particularly showing a set from the other master that he did not know well. This made the visiting master lose face, first through the "rudeness" of his student, secondly in not presenting his form to best advantage. Moral: never demonstrate in front of a master unless you are asked first and never demonstrate one master's form to another master unless you can do it flawlessly! Remember—Modesty!

Still one more example of Modesty—or the lack of such—comes to mind. In one of my classes I had a 6th degree Judo Black Belt who had trained for decades with some of the top Judo teachers in the world. A man of wide experience in martial arts, he had taught hand to hand combat and restraint techniques at numerous police academies. He was a wonderful Taiji player, who exuded martial spirit, tempered by restraint and great courtesy. In one class, I was teaching and demonstrating some basic Chin Na (joint locking) techniques, and planned to ask this student to demonstrate some of his much higher-level knowledge after I had finished.

Before that, students paired off and practiced. I noticed that my 6th degree Black Belt student happened to be paired off with a young "know-it-all" who constantly corrected and criticized his technique and told him all the reasons why it would never work. The master Judoist just smiled and gently applied each technique to the student.

During a break in the class, I called the student back into the studio office and told him about his training partner's stature in martial arts and that he could have easily "demolished" the student with just one simple maneuver. I admonished him to be more aware and courteous in the future.

On another occasion I had a student who did quite a lot of business in South Korea. He had virtually no proficiency in Taiji. Returning from a visit to Korea, he called me in great excitement to inform me that he had "defeated" a Korean Tae Kwon Do master in a sparring match. When I pressed him for details, he related how one of his Korean business associates had brought him to visit a very well known martial arts master, who was highly revered and who was a very advanced level practitioner at the head of his own school.

My student told me that when the master had asked him about Taiji, he proposed to the master that they "spar" a bit. The Master politely declined, but apparently my student was somewhat insistent, so finally the Master agreed to a "bout." According to my student, he very quickly was able to "neutralize" the master and unbalance him.

Hearing this rather amazing story, I told my student that he was an ignorant, arrogant fool. In order not to embarrass his friend, the businessman (who undoubtedly had great *guanxi* with the Master to even be allowed a visit), the Master agreed to the putative "bout," and quickly "allowed" himself to be defeated. The student was so abysmally ignorant, that he did not even realize that the Master considered him at such a low level, that he pretended to be "defeated." It showed the Master's quality as a martial artist of integrity, and the student's complete failure at understanding even the most basic elements of martial etiquette.

I immediately dismissed him from my school.

Guanxi

Cultivation of *guanxi* is more complicated. It is a relation of trust and regard for the other that is built up over time. While any student can learn "forms," the more internal teachings are usually reserved for students who have cultivated *guanxi*. This is done through unfailing courtesy to the teacher (more on this later), sincerity in practice, and helping the teacher in various ways. One example of *guanxi* came about when a new Chinese restaurant opened in town. One of my friends, an American professor of Chinese at a prestigious local college, ate there frequently because the food was excellent. The manager then asked the professor for his help in translating some legal contracts, etc., which the professor did willingly.

Thereafter, whenever the professor would go there to eat, he would be given the "royal treatment" with unusual dishes and impeccable service. This in turn would tip the delicate balance of *guanxi* in favor of the restaurant so they could count on the professor's help in the future. This kind of relating is subtly balanced. In inviting a master to dinner, for instance, one is already creating *guanxi* and the master may decline for precisely that reason. It may not be time yet to enter into a more than casual relation with a student.

American students are sometimes very puzzled, even deeply disturbed, when a Chinese teacher seems to distance them abruptly and without apparent reason. Often this occurs with the most devoted and sincere students, who have helped the master in many ways. Sometimes this is because the teacher feels the balance of *guanxi* is becoming too extreme toward the student and the teacher must withdraw to avoid creating even more *guanxi* in the student's favor. Remember that any time you offer to do anything special for the master or his family, you are creating relationship and the master may need to evaluate the precise extent of the relation that is being created.

The logical outcome of development in *guanxi* (to the Chinese mind) is that the student will begin to request inner teachings soon. And the teacher may feel that the proper time has not yet come.

When Professor Cheng Man Ch'ing studied with the great Taiji Quan master Yang Ch'eng Fu, he was already a well-known traditional Chinese physician. During the course of his time with Yang, Yang's wife became seriously ill and he prevailed upon the Professor for medical advice. When Cheng cured Yang's wife, this created tremendous *guanxi* and Yang then felt obligated to share some special teachings with the Professor. One very important matter is to always follow through on any promise or agreement given to your teacher. This is just common courtesy, but in Chinese terms, agreeing to do something for your teacher is creating *guanxi* and if you do not follow through, this is considered very disrespectful and actually creates negative *guanxi* for you. So it is better not to make any promises you can't deliver on.

Does all this sound very convoluted and complicated? Actually it is not, it is just common courtesy refined to a subtle level. Here are a few individual points of etiquette you should know:

Preliminaries:

When you first meet a master, prepare to become a beginning student again, regardless of your previous training. The master will discern your real level of training soon enough. It is very bad manners to request immediately to be put into an advanced class; let the master decide. I have always been amazed at the number of people who used to come to my classes, asking to be put into an advanced class after some very modest amount of previous training with another teacher. In such cases, I would first have the class "Hold the Moon" for about 30 minutes. Invariably, the "advanced" newcomers would find their legs shaking after about 3 minutes and would come to a realization about their real state of training.

With one teacher I studied in private sessions for 4 1/2 years "just" to learn 8 moves! It was an absolutely transformative experience.

At our very first meeting I realized this master's level and quality. I had practiced extensively for over nine years at the time of our meeting, but decided to "empty" myself and even become a total beginner again, if necessary. He asked me whether I wanted to learn "many forms" to impress my friends or to become a "real student." I opted for the latter. Those 4 1/2 years in which I learned "only" 8 moves changed my entire concept of training and had ramifications on every level of my practicing the forms I had learned in previous years.

Respect a Master's "Gifts"

I heard one story from a friend who was privileged to learn from a 91 year old "Immortal" on the Chinese mainland. My friend, an expert in Chinese courtesy, soon became the Master's first foreign disciple, and had the very singular honor of giving a speech (in English!) at the Master's funeral. One day a friend of his from the States visited the hilltop where they trained at dawn each day in a pavilion overlooking the Yangtze River. The friend watched the class for a while, then was asked by the Master to demonstrate a form. It is always something of a phenomenon to the Chinese when an American knows Taiji Quan. The Master was pleased with the visitor and asked him to come the next morning for some instruction.

The following day the Master left his other students, some of whom had been with him 20-30 years, and devoted more than an hour to the young American visitor, showing the initial moves of a sword form. After the class, as the two Americans descended the mountain path, the visitor said he didn't think the class was worth much because he'd never learn the rest of the form anyway. My friend was shocked..."Just being with such a master is a teaching; watching how he holds the sword, watching how he moves, how he observes you, how he teaches; is in itself invaluable! How can you say it isn't worth much?"

In a similar vein, one of my old-time students was going to a *qigong* seminar with a famous martial arts teacher and said he hoped it wasn't only about beginning meditations or postures such as "Holding the Moon." I replied that the real teaching was seeing what the teacher did with those postures, not the external forms themselves. How does the teacher use those forms creatively? What new can you learn from his approach? Always remain modest in the face of any real teacher; if you look deeply there is much you can learn.

Always speak respectfully of your former teachers. No real teacher will ever appreciate your bad-mouthing other teachers. As Master Liang always admonished, "Praise their good points; say nothing about their defects." Always speak modestly about your previous training and experience. If you are asked to join a class already in progress, go to the back of the studio and follow along as best you can. Do NOT do your own forms in the new teacher's class; try to follow what the class is doing.

I once had an old student who had gone on to study with another teacher and came back asking if he could join my class again. I said yes, and the student, right in the middle of my group, performed his Solo Form as he had learned it from the other teacher, with many different variations, timings, etc., causing a break in our energy flow, and confusion among some of my beginning students. Very bad etiquette indeed!

Lacking Appreciation and Missing a Great Opportunity

As a beginning student, when I had learned Karate for about 6 months in a branch school in the suburbs of Boston, my teacher asked me to go to the main *dojo* downtown (mentioned earlier) to pick up some books, but it had to be early in the morning, because the master left for his regular job at around 8:30 AM. I arrived there promptly at 6AM, before his class. After I had gotten the books, the master invited me to join the class with his Black Belt students. I said thanks anyway, but it was still early in the morning and I would rather go home and go back to bed. The master stood there aghast and simply said, "If you want to go to bed, you had better go to bed!" I knew immediately that something was very wrong, but it was considerably later before I realized the master was showing me an uncommon courtesy in letting me practice with his advanced students. Instead of gratefully accepting the "master's gift," I had really "blown it." Yes, this was the same master whose table I had sat on 6 months earlier! At this point I decided to study etiquette seriously...

Another time I had invited a well-known teacher to present a seminar at my school, teaching the "Sinew-Changing" exercises of the Shaolin School, attributed to Bodhidharma. An hour or so after the seminar began; I realized that I myself would never really be inclined to practice these exercises in my own daily training. I began to feel a bit frustrated, knowing I would spend the whole weekend learning a set of exercises that I did not intend to practice. It felt like a waste of time.

During a break, the teacher approached me, fully aware of what I was feeling. "Just take the whole experience as a blessing," he said. "If you receive it as a blessing, you will certainly get some gem of great value." Sure enough, I did. But more importantly, I never forgot that very wise advice—and have received many unexpected blessings ever since.

How to Behave as a Guest

Always accept graciously a teacher's invitation to join a class as a guest. When you are a guest in a class, it may happen that one of the students there is anxious to prove his skills against you (in

Push Hands). This is a delicate situation. Knocking down another teacher's student in their own studio is often regarded as a "loss of face" for that teacher and of an overly aggressive attitude on the part of the visitor. It is usually better to neutralize, but not really counter too strongly, to let your skills be shown without detriment to the other. The acme of skill, of course, is to effectively neutralize the other person's attacks, find their defects that you could use for an uproot and then just release energy ever so gently, causing a slight imbalance, but no obvious uproot or knockdown. Any master will immediately recognize this as a very high level of *kung fu* and ethical cultivation. You will bring honor, both to your teacher and yourself.

One of the great stories illustrating this degree of precision and control concerns Yang Lu Ch'an, founder of the Yang School. After studying Taiji Quan from the Chen Family for some 18 years, he made his way to Beijing and soon established himself as a leading martial arts master. In keeping with the custom of the times, he met many challenges and was never defeated. At one point a high-ranking prince (some stories say the Emperor himself) summoned Yang to demonstrate his skills. Yang was ordered to face the Prince's master boxing teacher in a match. A very delicate situation...If Yang were defeated, he might be regarded as a charlatan and banished from the city. But if he knocked down or injured the Prince's master boxer, he would cause tremendous loss of face to the Prince. As the master boxer attacked furiously, Yang simply neutralized each attack, without countering. At one moment, sensing an opening, he placed his fist gently on the master boxer's ribcage, then bowed and withdrew. It was obvious to all that he could have landed a disabling blow, but no one was injured, or even knocked down. The Prince's dignity was maintained intact and Yang's skills were shown at their highest level. This is the true acme of the art!

My friend who studied in China reported a similar experience. Some of the students of his 91 year old Master had been with the Master for over 30 years! Yet those students, who my friend said were superior to almost any "master" in the U.S., considered themselves only mid-level students. When my friend joined their class, he was the "foreign professor." When he would engage in Push Hands with the senior students, who were vastly more skilled than he was, he would often be maneuvered into an unstable position. Instead of uprooting him or knocking him down, the Master's student would say

"Oh, excuse me, I've made a mistake..." and not press his advantage. It was evident to all who was the more highly skilled, but my friend the "foreign professor" was not embarrassed in any way.

Remember that whenever you visit another teacher or school, you are a representative of your teacher. Any master will realize that you may not fully represent your teacher's expertise in form (though some students surpass their teachers), but you will definitely manifest your teacher's fundamental attitude. And, since practice of Taiji is devoted in large measure to cultivation of "temperament," many masters will look on your attitude as the real indicator of your accomplishment. A modest and restrained, yet centered attitude is best.

Going to Dinner

One of the surest ways in which *guanxi* is cultivated is in going to dinner with the Master and fellow students, often after class or seminars or on special holidays. Knowing even the rudiments of proper Chinese table etiquette will show great respect to your teacher. If you are going to a restaurant, it is good to reserve in advance, or pick out the appropriate table yourself. The best table is usually farthest from the door and the seat of honor is facing the main doorway. If you go regularly to the same restaurant with your teacher, the manager will eventually come to know you and will automatically provide the correct table, if it is available. Remember that cooking or operating a restaurant is one of the main avocations of martial arts masters and there is some chance that the cook or manager is himself a high level martial artist. If you all arrive at the restaurant together, let the Master be seated first in the seat of honor, then seat yourselves.

When tea is brought, fill the Master's cup immediately and keep it filled through the remainder of the meal; this is often done by one of the senior students who sits near the Master. After filling the Master's cup, the senior should fill everyone else's cup and keep an eye on the teacup situation. When the teapot is almost empty or the tea is cold, open the lid on the teapot and move the pot to the edge of the table, a traditional sign to the waiter to replenish the teapot.

When the food is brought, serve the Master first, then each person can take their own portion. Needless to say, there is also an art of ordering Chinese food, but that will be left for another article. [See my E-book: *"Nourishing Life, the Chinese Art of Healthy Eating.."* Available at www.totaltaichi.com]. When the meal is over, never let the Master pay for the meal. "The Master must never show his money." The students should contribute enough to cover the Master's meal and tip. Often the smoothest and most discreet way to arrange things is for the senior student to go and settle the bill shortly before the end of the meal and the others can settle with the senior outside or later on.

On occasion the Master will make a special point of treating the students, sometimes taking one or more out to a dinner with his family. In this case, if the Master insists on paying, accept graciously. Do not insist on paying yourself, since this will embarrass the Master. Just sense the flow of *qi* and everything will work out splendidly. If the Master is hosting a visiting master, the students should make sure that everything runs smoothly, and that the visiting master is honored in the appropriate way. This will reflect very highly on your teacher, as well as yourself.

One time I went to a demonstration given by a local master in Boston who had invited one of his brother classmates from a distant city to demonstrate with him. Though I was not a student of either master, I was a friend of one of the senior students. After the demonstration, the inevitable banquet followed, at one of the city's best Chinese restaurants. Several tables had been reserved in advance. I got there a bit early and saw immediately that there were two seats in the rear of the restaurant, facing the door, below an auspicious pair of Chinese characters adorning the wall. These were obviously the seats of honor. I sat near the door, since I was an outside guest and had no rank in that school.

After a short time, students began to come in and sat down in the seats of honor. I went over and told them these seats were the seats of honor, and should be reserved for the masters. The students graciously reseated themselves. A little while later, more students filtered in and again sat in the auspicious seats. Somewhat hesitantly, I went over again and told them about the proper etiquette for seating. They moved, but in a matter of moments the seats were filled again. This time I felt it was out of place for me to say more, so I remained at my table. Soon all the seats were filled up and the masters hadn't yet arrived. When the masters appeared, the host master immediately looked at the seats of honor, and I could see a dismayed expression flicker across his face. Not only were the seats of honor taken, there were no seats left at all! A most embarrassing situation! After some scurrying around by the manager, two seats were found and added to one of the long tables. The masters sat near the doorway and the students occupied the seats of honor!

When you are going to meet your teacher at a restaurant always be on time, even a bit early, if possible. You should be there to greet the Master, not the other way around. Once, after a very successful seminar, my students and I hosted T.T. Liang to a banquet. It was great. About sixty people showed up and all arrangements had been made in advance—excellent food, proper seating, etc. Since the Master had been running about 15 minutes late through the seminar and I was very busy with arrangements, I was still some distance from the restaurant at the time appointed for the banquet. Speeding into the parking lot, I found one my Old Timers who had come out to inform me that everyone, including the Master, was already seated. As I walked in, the Master looked up at me and with his deep and resonant voice said, "Oh, the Big Potato comes..." I felt like the "smallest potato" imaginable at that moment.

Other Important Points

Do not always ask for more knowledge, forms, etc. Let the teacher judge. The body must be molded correctly for progress to occur on a deep level. Learning "forms" is only the "skin and hair" of practice. Any good teacher will want to see that your forms have been internalized, and no good teacher will hold a willing student back unnecessarily. Let the teacher judge when the time is right for more knowledge to be imparted. Students should share the knowledge they have received freely with their brother and sister students who are at an equal level of study. However, it is not considered appropriate for a student to teach a lower level student more advanced material than that student has already learned from the teacher, unless the teacher has approved, or asked the student to teach it.

This is particularly true in the case of internal energy practices, meditations, etc. The body must be prepared inwardly for higher energy levels and this takes time. You are not benefiting a fellow student by teaching him/her advanced forms or internal techniques without the teacher's approval. A teacher must observe a student for some time to observe the student's capacity, attitude, etc. before showing some of the advanced knowledge. This is not for reasons of secrecy but for the student's own protection.

At one time I had a student who was very fascinated with books on esoteric Taoist meditations. He would bring one book in particular to class almost every week and ask for my advice on how to perform the complex meditations described in the book. The book was a translation of one of the most famous Taoist meditation texts from many centuries ago. The ultimate goal was to create a "spirit body" which could leave the physical body at will and roam the empyrean.

When my student asked for advice, I always strongly admonished him that the book might be interesting for historical study, but ON NO ACCOUNT should he attempt to duplicate the practices depicted in the book. I was very emphatic about this. First, all such books were originally meant for initiated devotees of the Taoist sect, who had prepared for the higher practices with years of apprenticeship and personal tutelage. Second, many such books contained deliberate errors, precisely so that non-initiates could not acquire the meditation techniques without a personal teacher.

This student, who was quite a ladies' man, also brought a girlfriend to the class almost every week. She was a lovely young college student, who would politely observe the class, or sometimes study in the back of the training hall. I thought she brought really pleasant energy to the class, even as a non-participant.

After becoming accustomed to her presence at the class, I noticed that she had been absent for several weeks, and casually asked my student how she was. He replied that she was "having a few problems." I asked him to give her my greetings and well-wishes. A few more weeks passed and she still had not returned as a visitor to the class. My student mentioned that she was "not feeling well," and again I asked him to give her my greetings.

A few more weeks went by and I asked the student how his friend was. He paused a bit then replied that she was in the state mental hospital. I was quite shocked and amazed, and asked for more details. He sheepishly mumbled that he had "gotten her up to chapter seven." I then realized that he had been trying to teach his friend the meditations from the book!

This experience gave me a whole new insight into why the esoteric teachings had been carefully guarded through the centuries — for the protection of students from their own ignorance!

Money

Most often in older times, martial arts instruction was available only after the student was recommended, personally interviewed, and accepted by the master. The student understood that study would be a long-term relationship with the teacher and fellow students. Quite often, the master would be employed by an extended family as a resident teacher and all of the master's and his family's needs would be provided. Outside students would often bring gifts of food or other necessities. Cash was not the usual medium of exchange. Still, no student would even think of accepting instruction without a return of some kind. At times, if a student did have cash, a master might be given a red envelope full of money. This would be considered more appropriate than simply handing cash directly. Some well-known teachers, even today, like to be given a financial token of respect in a red envelope. But this is not universal; other teachers (from different parts of China) consider red envelopes something that a superior would give to an inferior, since they are often given to children on Chinese New Year's Day. So the best policy is to check with fellow students to see if this mode of financial respect is acceptable to a given teacher. Most often in the States, masters accept cash payments, since this is much simpler than the old payments in kind and considerations of *guanxi*.

I personally don't know of any Taiji teacher who teaches principally for the money. Most often it is a matter of sharing an art which is beautiful to share. If you find that the fee for instruction is genuinely too expensive for you, tell the teacher what you can afford at the present time. I know of no teachers who will turn Taiji students away solely for lack of money. Just be honest and fair to your teacher and he or she will respond in kind. In traditional etiquette it would be considered extremely disrespectful to debate the cost of instruction with your teacher. Remember that the art you are learning is a lifetime gift leading to enhanced health, energy, longevity (possibly even "Immortality!"), and the making of many new friends. If you feel that the instruction is genuinely overpriced, however, look elsewhere.

If you visit another teacher or school, always pay for the class. If the teacher refuses, you can leave a small offering of tea, incense, etc. for the school. Also, when visiting your Master, always bring some small gift—fruit, tea, etc. This is a traditional sign of respect. Send a card or call your teacher on Chinese New Year's day. Treat fellow students from all schools as your Taiji brothers and sisters. Occasionally you may encounter someone with an aggressive attitude, but this is rare in Taiji circles. If this happens, remain centered and good humored, yielding as necessary.

Some Basic Terms

"Master" I reserve this word for someone who has not only reached a very high level in the physical aspects of the art, but in its moral and philosophical aspects as well. The Master has a deep insight into people and has a wide perspective on life. The Master is more than expert in a martial art; the Master has attained spiritual maturity and is "expert" in flowing through life, helping students and people in general on as many levels as possible. In the Far East, it is usually considered impossible to have attained this level of maturity before age 60. Many true masters refuse to be called "masters," preferring instead to be called teacher or guide.

" Teacher" Someone well versed in physical aspects of the art and who has demonstrated the ability to share knowledge effectively and selflessly with others. Anyone who teaches should be on a committed path of lifetime practice.

"Disciple" Someone who has entered the Master's family, usually at some sort of formal ceremony. A disciple is considered a son or daughter of the Master and, in old times, had filial responsibilities to the Master and his family. A disciple gets the full teaching of the art, with no reservation, since he is in a relationship of complete trust with the Master.

"Student" Anyone who signs up for classes. Students will be taught forms, some internal energy techniques, and whatever the teacher or master deems appropriate. The student has no formal responsibilities to the Master or his family. It is a lighter commitment on both sides.

How does all this apply in America? My view is that there are only a few genuine American masters at this time. Inner cultivation takes decades and we have simply not had time enough to fully incorporate the teachings. There are, however, many excellent American teachers. I would also say that it would be unusual, if not inappropriate, for a teacher to make "disciples," a practice traditionally reserved for masters. The entire concept of discipleship is foreign to most Americans and the obligations incurred, both to the Master's well-being and to propagating the art, may be too much for most American students to commit to.

In general, the American Taiji scene is characterized more by informality, sharing, and good will. This is our strength in the art. We can blend the best from various teachings, and even bring masters together to share their knowledge and further develop Taiji.

The basics of etiquette treated in this article are most relevant to interactions between American students and traditional Chinese masters. Most American teachers eschew the more formal older etiquette and not a few American teachers are completely ignorant of it and couldn't care less. Still, since they are at the root of much of the traditional teaching system, they are valuable knowledge for all students. In time, we will develop our own Taiji etiquette here in the States, a blend of traditional Chinese and American values. This process is already occurring. Meanwhile, some attention to the older standards of etiquette and *guanxi* will enrich your practice by providing a firm moral and psychological grounding to the physical aspects of your art.

For me, study of traditional Taiji courtesy is in itself a profound and subtle way to learn *qi* flow through human relations, a "Push Hands" of daily life, which enhances awareness and appreciation and reverberates through all areas of life.

At "Banquets" — How to Order Chinese Food

Lin Yutang, the famous Chinese scholar and writer of the 1940's and 50's once said that all of Chinese philosophy could be reduced to one good meal. (See his wonderful book *The Importance of Living*.) A connoisseur of fine food himself, Lin lived to be over 90. [This brief discussion of selecting Chinese dishes is greatly amplified in my E-book on *The Chinese Art of Healthy Eating*, referred to above.] The most basic distinction in Chinese nutritional science is between hot and cold foods. Since human life itself is characterized by heat—the warmth of red blood, circulation, digestion, and maintenance of body temperature, there is always a slight bias toward warmer foods. Warm foods are the meats and spicier dishes. Neutral foods are the grains. Cooler foods include vegetables and fruits. Some foods, such as tofu and sprouts, are particularly cold and are never eaten raw by the Chinese (who seldom eat raw foods anyway). In ordering Chinese food, it is best to have 4-8 people at the table, so that a greater number of dishes can be shared.

Depending on season and weather conditions, one can emphasize either colder or warmer dishes. In winter more spicy meat dishes are appropriate; in summer more dishes containing tofu, mushrooms, and vegetables. On hot summer days one can also eat cold noodles, or bean threads (which are extremely cooling). On damp days, one chooses a greater selection of spicy dishes, which cause sweat, thus dispelling damp from the body. However, in warm damp weather, these can be more vegetal in nature, or with more seafood. In general, chicken is mildly hot and benefits the kidneys, beef benefits the blood and spleen, lamb is very warm and builds body heat. Fish are colder and can be cooked with hot spices to remove some of their cooling quality, or more mildly to retain it. In summer, order mild seafood dishes; in winter you can order spicier ones. With a group of 4-8 people, one would generally order one dish from each category; one chicken, one beef, one or two seafood, and a couple of vegetable dishes.

I once was at a festive dinner in Boston Chinatown where 6 of the 8 people (all Americans) ordered chicken dishes. The owner, an elderly lady, came running over to our table, looked at us in disbelief, then began scolding us for all ordering the same category. That was one of my first introductions to Chinese dietetics. So order from a wide variety, taking into account appropriate amounts of spicy or mild dishes, according to people's tastes and weather conditions. A small amount of tea is drunk before the meal to enhance conversation and get digestive juices flowing. Though many people drink during the meal (if you need to drink a lot of tea, there is probably MSG in the food), it is generally advised to drink sparingly while eating so as not to reduce the digestive "fires." After the meal, a bit more tea can be taken to help reduce the effects of fats in the body.

For purposes of training *qi* cultivation, it is best to avoid deep-fried or overly greasy foods. The meaty dishes selected should contain a wide variety of vegetables. Avoid dishes which have thick sauces and a lot of salt or oil. Balance hot with cold, spicy with mild, colors, textures, and flavors. If you are alone, order a dish with slight amounts of meat or seafood and plenty of vegetables. Vegetarians can order hotter or cooler vegetal dishes in accordance with the season. Then enjoy the harmony and friendship of a good meal. You can learn Chinese philosophy, enhance *guanxi* and cultivate *qi*

Final Note

You may have heard the old expression, "Go to the teacher with an empty teacup." That is very true. But just make sure that your teacup is empty and the Master's is full!

Chapter 15

How to Find a Good Taiji Teacher

As "Tai Chi" becomes ever more popular in the United States and around the Western world, it is essential for a prospective student to understand how to select a truly qualified teacher. Without studying under a high-level teacher, you will gain only the most superficial results from your considerable investment of time, energy, and money.

As the Chinese say, you will get merely the "skin and hair" of the art, not the "bone and marrow." So if you want the "marrow" of the art, you must find a good teacher!

Essential Qualities Your Teacher Must Have

"Lineage"

The very first qualification any good Taiji teacher must have is a lineage. That means that the teacher can demonstrate a line of succession that goes from him/her back to a recognized Style of Taiji Quan, and ultimately, to the founder of that Style.

There are several common Styles of Taiji Quan practiced in the United States:

> **The Yang Style**, standardized by Yang Ch'eng Fu in the 1920's, and the derivative "Yang Style Short Form" created by Cheng Man Ch'ing.

> **The Wu Jian Quan Style**, standardized by Wu Jian Quan and Ma Yueh Liang.

> **The Chen Style**, derived from Chen Zhang Xing, with several current lineage holders, among them Chen Xiao Wang and Feng Zhi Chiang.

> **The Sun Style**, established by Sun Lu Tang and standardized by him and his daughter Sun Jian Yun.

And a few lesser known Styles, including the traditional **Taoist Wu Dang Style** and the **Yang Mi Quan Style**, as well as the newly-created **"Twenty Four"** and **"Forty Eight"** Movement Styles, which were created by modern "Sports Committees" in China.

The purpose of this chapter is not to delve into the history of the various Taiji Quan Styles and families, since that would require an entire book to do it justice. Rather, it is simply to indicate that any teacher of quality can show that his/her art is genuine and derives from a recognized Style of the art. For a fascinating partial history of Taiji Quan's development see *Lost T'ai-chi Classics from the Late Qing*

Dynasty by Professor Douglas Wile. Also, note the excellent brief history written by Scott Rodell and available on his website at **www. grtc.org**

Finding a real teacher is absolutely critical in the current Taiji environment in the United States where there are a number of master-level teachers of very high achievement, but there are also numerous "teachers" who have taken only a few classes, or even just one seminar. Many "teachers" teach self-created movement awareness techniques and breathing exercises and call it "Tai Chi." Other teachers combine Yoga, Taiji, dance, and body awareness exercises and label that "Tai Chi."

Just be aware that in order to glean the genuine health and body-mind development benefits of Taiji Quan, you MUST learn the genuine art from a real teacher. As the Taiji Classic, "Song of the Substance and Function of the Thirteen Forms" says: "If you do not seek carefully [study according to the principles of the *Taiji Quan Classics*] and examine thoroughly, your time and effort will be spent in vain, and you will have cause to sigh with regret." That also means that your teacher must be well versed in the *Taiji Quan Classics* and teach according to the principles in the *Classics*. That is the only true art of Taiji.

I once had a woman in my brand new beginners' class who informed me that she had "32 people waiting" for her Taiji class which would begin the very next day! When I asked what her previous level of training had been, she said she had had NO training whatsoever. She had come to my class to learn something she could teach to her class the following day.

At first I was quite sure I had misunderstood, but when it became obvious that she had indeed had NO previous Taiji training, I was simply speechless in shocked amazement.

That is, of course, a very extreme example. But be sure to check your prospective teacher's lineage, as well as how long they have been actively training under their teacher. Remember the old martial arts proverb:

> *"One hundred days, small accomplishment*
> *One thousand days, middling accomplishment*
> *Ten thousand days, great accomplishment."*

That means at the very least that your teacher should have about three years of formal training and daily study before teaching. And this is the absolute minimum requirement. At the other extreme, your teacher may have almost 28 years of training, which would be excellent.

One final point regarding the age of your teacher: It is a Chinese tradition that a "teacher should not be too young or too old." Too young means their art and experience of life is still immature; too old means that they may be unable to fully demonstrate the techniques. In general, the best masters are said to be between 45 and 75 years old. But there are exceptions. Some teachers are remarkably proficient and mature even at a young age, while others can be in advanced years and still in excellent condition to demonstrate the entire art of Taiji. So just find out the lineage and experience level of a teacher before beginning to study.

Knowledge of the Taiji System

Of the entire "universe" of Taiji Quan teachers in the United States, only a small fraction know the entire Taiji System. When most Americans think of Taiji, what they imagine is the slow-moving Solo Form. They do not realize that Taiji is a multi-faceted art, which includes numerous elements for a complete and all-encompassing method of mind-body training. You can look at Chapter 13 in this book, "The Taiji System" for more details.

The important point when selecting a teacher is that a teacher at least be aware that there IS a Taiji System. If your prospective teacher thinks the Solo Form is all of Taiji, look elsewhere. It is not necessary for your teacher to actively know or be proficient in every facet of the Taiji System, but s/he should at least understand the rudiments of two-person work (Push Hands and defensive Applications), and preferably know one or more weapons forms (Saber and Sword are most commonly practiced).

If the teacher you are interviewing has "no clue" about Taiji defensive Applications and weapons, their teaching will lack any depth and real understanding.

Your own aspiration in Taiji will determine the level of teacher with whom you should study. If you simply want basic physical fitness and relaxation, a low level teacher may suffice. But if you want to truly experience the deeply rejuvenating effects of Taiji or want to learn Taiji Quan as a martial art, a high level teacher is absolutely essential. While Taiji is widely renowned as a profoundly effective healing art, its truly remarkable health benefits can only be achieved if it is taught and studied correctly.

Of the recent generation of grandmasters, Professor Cheng Man Ch'ing cured himself of tuberculosis by Taiji Quan; T.T. Liang was deathly ill in his early forties, began serious practice of Taiji, and lived to be 102; Master Jou Tsung Hua had a heart ailment in his late forties and totally cured himself, becoming "younger" and more vigorous each year until his untimely death in a car accident in his early eighties. And similar stories apply to Masters Benjamin Lo and Abraham Liu.

So Taiji Quan is truly an art of deep physical rejuvenation and "immortality." But to get these benefits, you must study seriously with a high level teacher.

Teaching Methods

Needless to say, teaching methods differ widely. You should find a teacher whose methods accord with your own temperament and willingness to learn.

In general, I would recommend avoiding any teacher who uses coercion and intimidation while teaching. While a strict, no-nonsense approach is to be desired, no teacher should demean or intimidate a student. And if the teacher insists you follow every Form s/he teaches like a robot, or claims that their version of the "Form" is the one and only genuine Taiji, I would respectfully depart and look elsewhere.

In the beginning, students need to get a sound foundation and structure and that temporarily entails following (or mimicking) every detail of the teacher's Form. But once students have mastered the basics, they must evolve to discovering their own optimal "flavor" of the Form, which fully suits their particular physical abilities and temperament. Much like playing music and following a musical score, students will practice the genuine "Form," but their "flavor" or personal interpretation depends upon their age, body type, temperament, etc.

I am always amazed by young students who studied with an 80 year old teacher and perform the "80 year old's Taiji Form." It looks quite silly! Sometimes these students are quite resistant to hearing that, as young players, their movements should be more stretched out with deeper stances. After all, they say, their Master did a very conservative, understated, high form. When they come to realize that the Master, over maybe a 50 year period, gradually internalized and minimized his/her Form, it makes sense to them not to slavishly copy a "Form," but to use the Principles to create their own essence in Taiji.

A good example of this came years ago when I studied with the late B.P. Chan, a most meticulous and painstaking teacher, who would correct every nuance of a student's movements. I had studied with him for about 3 years when I came to my private class one day and asked him to correct one of my moves, which just didn't feel quite right. He retorted, "Find out for yourself." At first I was a bit surprised and just thought he might be out of sorts on that particular day. So I practiced alone for a while then asked again if he could correct the move. This time he said, "You figure it out."

By now I was quite miffed, since I had commuted some 4 hours one-way to come to the lesson, and paid what was then a substantial amount of money to me as a young student. Chan perceived my level of upset, and quietly said, "Your *qi* is your teacher now. You must find out the correct movement from inside. My showing you won't help anymore." So at first, a new student's Form must be acquired by imitating the teacher, but as progress comes, the student must find his/her own way.

One other matter concerning teaching methods is important. Taiji is the art of YIN and YANG. That means, Taiji should seek to create the perfect BALANCE in the student's body and personality. Many American teachers teach only to "relax, relax, relax!" I believe this is not always beneficial to the student. Although some of the legendary older masters in China (Yang Ch'eng Fu as an example) are said to have taught by admonishing students to "relax," one must remember that often students of these well-known masters had had years or even decades of previous martial art training. They had a firm structure, a "root," and could project tremendous power.

So the teacher's job was to show them how to internalize that power and use it more efficiently. That is—the student was to go from an overly Yang state to a slightly more Yin state to create overall balance.

But in America today the vast majority of Taiji students are already much too Yin. They lack structure, "root," and often lack energy. Yet they are taught to "relax!" In this case, the teacher should give them rooting and structural exercises to begin to develop their internal strength and create a base of Yang energy. Look for a teacher who is versatile and knowledgeable enough to adopt, Yin OR Yang teaching methods to meet a student's needs. And at best, find a teacher who knows how much information to teach at an appropriate level to the students' development.

I have seen teachers teaching rank beginners, who are attempting to show them sophisticated Applications, or who are giving greatly excessive detail. Remember, it is not how a much a teacher "knows," but the amount a student can assimilate at any given time that is the key to effective teaching.

Atmosphere During Class

When scouting out a prospective Taiji teacher, always request to visit a class. There are a very few teachers who may refuse such a request, but if they do, Caveat Emptor! When you do go to observe a class, the atmosphere should be serious, focused, yet devoid of tension or stress. The students and teacher should appear happy and in good spirit.

Most Taiji schools have a fairly relaxed external discipline compared with other martial arts schools. That is, there is no bowing, commands yelled out, or a sense of military discipline. There should be at atmosphere of quiet ease, yet serious intent. I remember a visitor at one of B.P. Chan's classes. He had been quite experienced in other martial arts and wanted to "check out" Chan. After the class, he approached Chan and mentioned that the class didn't seem too disciplined. Chan paused a moment, then said, "Here we don't worry too much about 'outside'; we just take very good care of 'inside.'"

Just as you should avoid a Taiji school characterized by severe external discipline, you should also avoid a school where a lax atmosphere prevails. Too much standing around, talking, or a teacher who explains endlessly or spouts "fortune cookie wisdom" is a bad sign. Practice and refinement is essential and that should be the focus of the class.

In the end, provided your prospective teacher has a Lineage and enough experience to teach effectively and honestly, much will be revealed by your own gut feeling. Remember, you and the teacher should be in resonance for the alchemy of profound learning to be achieved. But don't confuse resonance with being a "pal" of the teacher. You want a teacher who can effectively motivate you and challenge you to your best level of achievement, not a "Taiji buddy."

References

After you have visited a class, discreetly ask some of the students their opinions and experiences with that teacher. Also, you might check well-known listings of Taiji teachers at **http://scheele.org/lee/tcclinks.html.** Or seek advice from the editors at *Tai Chi* magazine. Often experienced martial artists of other traditions can also offer a valuable critique of your prospective Taiji teacher.

Professional ethics

It should go without saying that a teacher should demonstrate a high level of professional ethics. A teacher should not exploit his/her students, constantly asking them to do favors or errands. Some assistance to and respect for the teacher is appropriate and an excellent way to create *guanxi* (see chapter on "Chinese Etiquette.") But if the teacher is constantly asking for favors or imposing tasks out of class, they are probably exploiting the students.

Also, if the teacher has students teach most of the classes, this is not a good sign. Senior students can and should assist the Teacher in correcting beginning students or helping with classes, but if the Teacher is never around and seems to have students teaching all or most of the classes, move on. This is simply a way to increase enrollment and save the Teacher's energy. But you want the majority of your instruction to come from the Teacher him/herself, not an assistant.

As was mentioned earlier, any cruel or sadistic treatment of the students during class is absolutely unacceptable. Likewise, be very wary about a teacher who has any sexual involvements with students.

A teacher should be able to really listen to the student as well as teach. The teacher should demonstrate a genuine care for students and that means finding out what the students' real needs are.

Finally, when a teacher feels that the student has really assimilated all of his/her knowledge, the teacher must be able to "let go," and allow the student to go on to another teacher. And the teacher should welcome a student's exploration of other teachers and styles. While it is necessary to be devoted to just one teacher and Style until your base is firmly established, at some point you will want to explore other areas and flavors of study. A good teacher will encourage this; lesser teachers will be offended or upset.

One of T.T.Liang's wonderful points is that he would encourage students to explore other teachers and styles, then when they came back, Liang would take the new forms or information and "make it Taiji's way."

The exploration for and finding a good Taiji teacher can be an exciting experience in itself. It will broaden your horizons and knowledge base, and hopefully connect you with the perfect teacher to teach you the beautiful art of Taiji, "to retard old age and make Spring eternal."

Chapter 16

Taoist Tales

Original stories by the "recluse of Wu Ming," now said to be dwelling somewhere to the South.....

These short stories embody much ancient Taoist lore. In the now extinct Chinese "old style" culture, there was much allusion and play on names. In Taoism there was often a kind of exaggerated politeness in conversation and manners, all of which is reflected in the stories.

And the many embedded allusions in these Tales will provide a fertile ground for your personal research, if you so choose.

The tales depict a period in which family and martial arts lineage was paramount. Hopefully, they will entertain you, as well as introduce some little-known dimensions of the deeper levels of training

"Night Stroll at Hollow Valley"

(or, "The True Meaning of T'ai Chi")

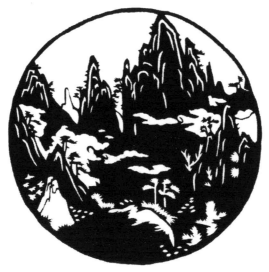

To my Tao-friend Laughing Cloud Monk,
Master of "nothing special"
and to the many wayfarers at Wu Ming.

Spring 1980

Night Stroll At Hollow Valley

Late afternoon in early May...I had been traveling since morning along gently rising foothills into the mountainous parts of Shanxi. A glorious day! Fields resplendent with brilliant green; peasants planting millet and vegetables; occasionally groups of children and dogs frolicking along the dusty roads, gazing curiously at the "Western Ocean Devil"—a strange green-eyed, white faced creature attired in Chinese black trousers and light blue tunic, a good outfit for journeying. Now, about an hour before sunset, the air took on that distant crystalline quality so conducive to meditation and inner quiet; the subtly mellowing color of gold-red sun turned the world into a terrestrial reflection of the Buddhist Pure Land in the Western Heaven. Peasants began appearing along the road talking and laughing, their day's labors done. They directed questioning glances toward me, but seemed to know that I had set forth on a specific mission, knew my destination, and had a sense of the lay of the land.

Soon the birds began their evensong, which always occurs shortly before sunset, the haunting melodies a real gift for a sensitive ear, and I too thought it time to express thanks to the great Way for the beauties of the day past. There was a small pavilion several hundred yards from the road, surrounded by cypress trees that had begun to sway in the gentle breezes of nightfall. Roads were deserted now. I could imagine the farmers enjoying their evening meal, and indeed smoke was wafting up from many huts. The pavilion was old and in need of paint, though traces of red lacquer were still visible on the pillars, and the place seemed to breathe an atmosphere of repose, as though travelers had paused to rest and refresh themselves there for many generations. A few verses were chiseled into the stone foundation, the characters now almost indecipherable, worn smooth by winds and rain. One line emerged clearly from the dusky rock,

"*The wise traveler, at leisure, gazes northwest...*"

A rather cryptic pronouncement. I thought it better to rest my legs and sip some mild wine than to ponder ancient mysteries.

Chanted the Heart Sutra and several chapters from the *Tao Te Ching*, then sat down to enjoy some lightly scented herbal wine and a few rice cakes before moving on. Lines of an old poem came to mind as a faint touch of evening damp began to pervade the air....

> *For about thirty years I wandered,*
> *Searching for the real Tao everywhere.*
> *How many times did I see the trees*
> *Grow new branches and watch the old leaves fall.*
> *But at this moment, seeing the peach blossoms,*
> *I am suddenly enlightened and have no more doubts.*

[Wang Wei, Author's translation]

Sipping wine, feeling very comfortable and rested, I gazed to the north of the line of the setting sun. A strange hollow in the hills seemed to arrest my eye—nothing spectacular, but the slight gap in the row of hills gave the entire range a special harmony. Though little detail could be discerned, my eyes seemed riveted to the place as though a magnet beam were drawing them there. It seemed curious.

"So, you have discovered the truth of our old poet's observation?" I looked around startled and somewhat annoyed at this interruption of my reverie. A dignified figure stood behind me, smiling slightly with a roguish expression in his eyes. He appeared to be a Taoist priest in his dark blue long gown, and his pleasantly rosy face was framed by the proverbial white beard. I looked perplexed, not quite sure of the significance of his question. My discomposure seemed to amuse him greatly, for his smile broadened and he looked beyond me into the hollow of the hills. I understood. *"The wise traveler, at leisure, gazes northwest..."* Rising to my feet I faced him and made a low bow. "Well, our guest from the Western Ocean is indeed a man of courtesy," said he, returning my greeting with a bow slightly lower than my own. "Allow me to introduce myself. For some time now, since I've taken to a traveler's life, people have addressed me as Zi-Jin Dao Ren, Purple Gold Taoist. Most likely I have been named so because of my great fondness for wandering these hills during the hours of sunset. And with whom have I the honor of being acquainted?"

"Your Reverence, this voyager from beyond the Western Ocean has several Chinese names, but prefers to be addressed as Jin-An, the one who makes peaceful progress like the sun rising over the earth."

"So, Jin-An, is it? A splendid cognomen indeed, and may I ask whence you have received such an honorable appellation?" I began to tell him of my coming to China some twelve years ago, but he gently looked beyond me into the hills again and said quietly, "Forgive me, Jin-An, but now is the time to follow the gaze of our ancient unknown friend and poet; if you look closely you may perceive something of interest in the hollow of the hills." I peered into the deepening dusk. The gap in the hills appeared to be catching the last rays of the departing sun, though nothing nearby showed any traces of direct sunlight. Zi-Jin stood altogether impassive, as if mesmerized by some vision, and I continued looking out. We must have stood for a considerable time; presently awareness grew that the spot to the northwest still seemed to show traces of sunset luminance, but the entire valley around us was quite shrouded in the gathering early-summer twilight. A sort of peculiar sweet radiance seemed to be emanating from the place, like the light of an exceptionally long enduring sunset. Squinting, I tried to discern the precise nature of this puzzling radiance. To no avail! The more intently I looked, the less it appeared, until I discovered that only by allowing my eyes to rest gently upon the place could I continue to perceive the delicate glow.

A slightly muffled giggle surprised me and I noticed Zi-Jin turned slightly in my direction. "You see, dear Jin-An, it was not for naught that our ancient comrade chiseled his poem into the stones of this pavilion, though, sad to say, the rest of the poem has been effaced by the winds of time, as must be the case with all manifestations of Tao. How much more wisdom must have been borne away by the spring breezes and autumn rains...But I see you too have discovered the light in the hills. Shall I say more?" I nodded, and we sat down. He produced some dried fruits from the folds of his gown and we shared a simple meal. He seemed pleased with my wine, winking now and then over the wine cup.

"Forgive me, esteemed guest, for offering you such meager fare, but I myself eat very little solid food these days; the clear air of these mountains seems to nourish this old body quite satisfactorily. A bowl of rice every now and then and some tea or herbal wine keeps this old recluse anchored to the earth until time for my return to Tao, so I seldom carry provisions on my wanderings. Could you now tell me of your journey here? You seem a man deeply versed in our lore and life and you are obviously no mere tourist."

I was still looking off into the hills, feeling just a bit tired and mellowed by the wine. "Your Reverence, allow me to ask you about the strange light we just saw; my own story is not long, nor very interesting, and I beg to tell you in detail come morning."

"Very well, young guest, it does appear that you will be nodding off at any moment. So let me tell you briefly about the Hollow Valley. For well nigh one thousand years now the place you saw nestled into the distant hillside has been the abode of the Hollow Valley Hermit."

"What?" I sat bolt upright, forgetting for a moment the elegant diction of Taoist politeness, "Are you saying that a hermit has lived there for a thousand years?"

"Of course," he said, smiling mischievously as though at some private joke, "though not the same hermit, or at least different transmogrifications of one or more Immortals. Since early Sung one Hollow Valley Hermit after another has inhabited that place. Some have been trained there; others have come from afar and have made the place their own. Though there is no formal succession, we Taoists all know when the proper person has come to carry on the tradition and there is tacit approval given to the one who finally becomes the dweller of Hollow Valley. We all consider it a very sacred place."

All tendencies to sleep had now left me; I was stirred by a sudden strange interest. "Could we go and visit him? Perhaps he is the one whom my old Teacher in Beijing told me about, though my Teacher gave him no name. He only said that if I came west I might find a hermit who could instruct me, one who dwelled not far from the setting sun."

"Dear guest, few go to visit him, for he most often disappears into the mountains when visitors appear. If you like, you may travel there; it is but a few hours' walk. I myself have had the privilege of visiting him upon several occasions, but, not wishing to importune him further, cannot accompany you at this time. He seldom receives even Chinese visitors, and whether or not he has ever been host to a Western Ocean dweller is unknown."

I noticed that he used the expression "Western Ocean dweller" instead of the more familiar and common "Western Ocean demon," a name I had come to accept and even like in a perverse sort of way.

"Indeed the evening grows chill," he said, drawing his gown tighter around him, "and as I have no fixed abode, I cannot offer you hospitality for the night." I assured him that this was quite all right; I was used to sleeping in the open (though this was a peculiar thing to do by Chinese standards) and that I felt comfortable most anywhere. "Very well, dear friend, for I now feel that you may be an old companion from some previous existence here. Allow me to commune with Tao before drifting off to the dream palace of the Immortals. Perhaps it will be our good fortune to converse again at greater length tomorrow."

It took little time to prepare my bedding; hard sleeping surfaces didn't bother me and my padded quilt was sufficient for the mild evenings of May. I lay down, watching the stars through the open sides of the pavilion. On the other side of the octagonal wooden floor Purple Gold sat upright in meditation, his dark-robed figure slowly merging into the blackness of the night.

Fresh scent of early morning dew-air, that very special elixir of atmosphere before dawn, seemed to expand my lungs and bring me back to consciousness. It had been a very good sleep, unbroken by dreams, though I felt some regret at not accompanying Purple Gold to the dream palace of the Immortals. I looked over to where his figure had been the night before, wondering if he was still communing with Tao. Maybe he was, but his physical form had vanished. Just the primeval pre-dawn light that betokened a clear day and the cypresses beginning to stir and rouse themselves. I was rather surprised and disappointed by my "host's" abrupt departure, until I realized that his disappearance may have been a polite way of urging me more quickly upon my way. Pre-dawn travel would be especially joyous on so fine a May morning and, since he was not going to visit the Hollow Valley, we both would have had to linger if I had told him the tale of my travels. Onward! It took no time at all to fold my quilt, shoulder my pack, and be on my way.

I felt no hunger; perhaps Zi-Jin had been right. The air here <u>was</u> wonderfully clear and seemed imbued with a nutritive quality. The birds had not yet begun to sing greetings to the sun; walking was most invigorating in the cool air. The hill-gap seemed less pronounced in the daylight than it had been at dusk, but the road was clearly headed in the right direction, and I strolled on unconcerned.

Memories...My journey to the Middle Kingdom twelve years ago after a youth and education in New England . An abiding interest in things Chinese and adventures of the spirit. How far away it all seemed now on that small dirt road in rural China. Arrival in Beijing, my good fortune at securing a post as English tutor to advanced students at Bei Da University, a job that provided for my frugal needs, while allowing much free time to pursue other interests. Wandering the streets of the old Capital, enjoying the brisk clear sound of true "Mandarin," studying the Classics and poetry with venerable professors steeped in the old traditions. Then an introduction to the great White Cloud Monastery, first experiences with a teacher on the Way—studies of Taoist movement arts and medicine. The years flew by—summers spent traveling through the south and west. China, the vast, the ancient, the ineffable...Much joy in learning, but a few areas always unfulfilled—what was the spirit of the ancients who practiced Tao? How and why did they create such arts as Taiji and Ba Gua? What did they feel about life; how did they perceive the movement of Tao in their own bodies and minds? And how could I bring this understanding (once rediscovered) to the Land Between Two Oceans, an understanding still living and vibrant, but clearly destined to fade as China turned more to the ways of the West? Several times I asked my Teacher at White Cloud. Answer—a smile. Finally—more intense questioning: a demand for an answer.

An unforgettable afternoon on an autumn day in the old Northern Capital...we sat in his little courtyard, the waning sun still warming the ancient stone table at which we sipped fragrant Jasmine tea. He seemed pensive, occasionally eyeing me over his tea cup.

"Dear young friend in Tao, for I can hardly call myself teacher. Indeed, we are all voyagers on the Great Way itself, some younger, some older, but each of us a complete and perfect manifestation of Tao. I know well of your concern, your questions. But can any answer be given to the true questions of Life? I cannot give you any true answer, for all true answers can come only from the three great teachers—Heaven, Earth, and our deepest inner heart. Did not our old Master Lao-Tze say, *"The way that can be made into a way is not the Eternal Way?"* How then should I try to pass on to you a way? You are already a dedicated traveler, and in time the Way will appear of itself, as it does to all who are sincere." Pausing to gaze fondly at the blossoming chrysanthemums, yellow, red and gold, he inclined his head toward me slightly, as if to divine my reaction to his reply.

"Thank you, Reverend Teacher," I replied, "Truly what you say is correct and you have taught me far beyond what I may have deserved. Yet I do still feel an emptiness, an unanswered question. I know much about the techniques of meditation, of your ancient arts of Taoist practice, yet it seems my understanding must ever remain incomplete until I comprehend thoroughly the true spirit of the wise ones of old who first developed such arts as Taiji. How did they come to have such understanding? What did they feel; how did they live? Can any reply now be given to such queries, or is this understanding lost forever in the forgotten mists of time?"

"Ah, Jin-An," (it was he who had given me this name) "you were always one to probe deeply and so it is meet for a seeker of the Way. But do not forget that wisdom can only ripen in its own time, and ripeness is all. No answer from outside will be truly of an avail; and, as for the spirit of the ancients, it still lives , but we ourselves may have to become ripe in years before our inner light dawns." Another pause while he refilled his cup and I enjoyed the fine clear deep blue of Beijing autumn sky, the swallows darting about the rooftops, the play of light and shadow upon the hoary moss-covered stones near the fishpond, occasional fallen leaves drawn up by a whirlwind near the walls and spiraling across the courtyard. "I feel that the time of our parting may not be far off. You have studied well here and given me much joy as a guide along the Path. What you have already learned will become an ever-richer gift as your life proceeds, for understanding of the Way is capable of endless enlargement. The mysteries of Tao can only come to realization in their own time, and never to those in haste. When you travel west, seek one who dwells not far from the setting sun; he may possibly help to dispel your doubts." He emptied his cup, winked at me while pointing to the swallows, and strolled away across the yard.

The scene faded. Here I was; birds now singing in all their glory, praising the rising sun; farmers emerging from houses and walking briskly into the fields; wives standing in doorways, children clinging to their knees as the strange white-faced traveler passed by. I was beginning to work up an appetite; the hills seemed fairly close by now, not more than two or three hours away, if I could maintain my present pace. I decided not to pause for breakfast, but to reach the hollow before the onset of late morning's heat. Besides, there were few wine shops [small local eateries] in these rural districts and I had passed the last town of consequence early yesterday afternoon.

The road became dusty as I trudged on; the mountain gap, now considerably changed in perspective, seemed not much closer than it had been at dawn. I sat down under a wayside tree to rest and sip wine. Some farmers in white short-sleeved blouses and knee length black trousers were approaching on the road. Coming abreast of my tree, they paused momentarily, apparently wondering whether or not to address me in Chinese. "Good morning, I am a traveler from the Western Ocean regions. Could any of you gentlemen show me the way to the gap in those near mountains called the place of the Hollow Valley?" Their eyes lit up in astonishment at hearing me speak their language, and their faces relaxed into smiles.

"Old Sir, Hollow Valley is a place none of us have yet ventured to visit. It seems Immortals live there, and strange lights are seen in those parts at dusk. However, if you really want to go there, the road forks in about a mile; take the lesser path to the west." Though their directions were given in Shanxi dialect, they seemed clear enough, so I thanked them, and they moved on down the road.

After half an hour's rest I felt thoroughly refreshed; still had enough wine left for one rest stop and hoped I would not need it before reaching my destination. Billowy white clouds now began to form above the hills. As often happened, poems came to mind while I walked, and I quietly chanted them as I went on my way....

> *In my middle years I knew something of Tao*
> *and finally settled on south mountain.*
> *When the spirit moves,*
> *I wander alone amid beauties that only I know...*
> *I will walk till the waters end.*
> *Then sit and watch the rising clouds,*
> *And perchance meet an old man of the woods,*
> *And talk and laugh and never return.*
>
> *Where is the Temple of Accumulated Fragrance?*
> *For many miles, I enter cloudy peaks.*
> *Ancient trees, no paths of men;*
> *Mountain deep, somewhere a bell...*

The spring's sound swallows perilous rocks,
The sun's color is cool on the green-blue pines.
Dusk at the bend of an empty pool—
Quiet meditation subdues the poison dragon.

[Wang Wei, Author's translation]

Soon I came upon a fork in the road with a small altar and Buddhist shrine. A surpassing image of Kuan Yin was carved on its side. I bowed and took the path on the left, since I had been heading north. A short walk and the path began to rise; the dust of the road and open clarity of the fields gave way to thick foliage, still showing the vibrant green of spring. There was a smell of moist earth and many singing birds—more and more a mountain atmosphere. I had lost sight of the hill gap, but expected to find it when I reached the top of the ridge to which the path seemed directed.

Within an hour, after a strenuous climb, the path delivered me onto the top of a ridge from which I could see the entire range of hills. I decided it was time to finish my flask of wine. I could see a hut and garden, surrounded by gnarled old pines, across from me on another ridge tucked into the hillside. Hollow Valley! Enthusiastically polished off the wine and set out forthwith. Walking around the ridge took another several hours and as late afternoon came on, I arrived.

Approaching cautiously, not certain about my reception by the Hollow Valley Hermit (if he was indeed there), I made my way slowly through the thinning trees of the hillside to the edge of a medium-sized garden with several tea bushes in bloom. There was a palpable serenity about the place; everything seemed clear, almost luminous, and the flowering shrubs and trees glowed in the afternoon sunlight. There seemed to be no one about and I stood by the garden hesitating to go nearer the house. Finally I summoned enough courage to walk up to the gray stone hut with curving roof, whose steel-blue tiles contrasted nicely with the vermilion doorway and painted columns flanking the door. I knocked discreetly, yet loudly enough to be heard throughout the hut by anyone present. No answer. I decided to go to the farther side of the garden and sit on a large flat stone near some fragrant herbs. I drew a volume of poems from my knapsack and began to look them over, though by this time most of them had long since penetrated my memory.

I awakened to a gentle rustling sound behind me. It was shortly before sunset. A man of average height clad in a long gray gown was approaching from behind the house, carrying a bundle of leafy sprigs. His black hair was drawn into a bun on top of his head and he looked quite youthful, though there was a nobility in his bearing and gait that bespoke a man of mature years. I fancied he seemed just a trifle shy, as is sometimes true of people who rarely see other humans, or who have deliberately cloistered themselves. He paused slightly and I felt a stir of embarrassment at having come thus unannounced to his retreat. Since it was now close to sundown and his hut was quite far removed from other habitation, he could hardly do me the discourtesy of sending me away for the night, yet he was clearly a man not accustomed to entertaining. I rose and bowed low in greeting. He returned my bow and continued coming slowly toward me, looking steadily. I experienced no discomfort under his scrutiny, but I knew he was taking the measure of my character.

"Well, my good young friend, I see my old wandering companion Purple Gold has contrived to arrange your arrival at this negligent mountain hut at precisely the hour of sunset." I was stunned and just looked at him agape, but he continued with a puckish grin twitching at the corners of his mouth. "Yes, I had a feeling Purple Gold was up to some of his old tricks. Today he has sent me a guest. Is your name not Jin-An, the one who makes peaceful progress like the sun coursing over the earth? Then why hasten here all a-fever to visit this old hill-dweller who cannot even provide you a decent night's lodging and a suitable meal?"

I couldn't quite believe what I was hearing; it was impossible to imagine that Zi-Jin had traveled all the way here just to inform him of my coming, and I was quite sure that Zi-Jin really had no intention of visiting Hollow Valley at this time. I was about to reply, but he went on, "Yes, I am the one commonly referred to as the Hollow Valley Hermit, though many have borne the name before me. I am merely one of countless wayfarers who have dwelt in this place. For now let us maintain silence and eat an evening meal, poor though it may be. I am not much given to conversation these days and since we are both acquainted by name, little more need be said. I know why you have come here and we will talk a bit later on."

My initial astonishment and discomfort ebbed away as we entered the cool stone hut. He showed me to a pleasant room that faced southeast. There was a straw bed and a fresh looking flowered quilt. A few tea cups lined the shelves, their sides worn smooth by many hands, also a copy of Lao Tze's *Tao Te Ching*, the *I Ching*, and a few other Taoist texts. Before long I smelled food and, expecting that he would not summon me himself, entered the kitchen. We enjoyed a silent supper as the sun lowered itself behind the trees—rice and fresh herbs as well as a few mushrooms that seemed to be cooked in a special wine sauce. This latter dish appeared to please my host especially; he looked up while eating it, smiled at me, and proffered the bowl, as if asking me to take more. We soon finished; I helped wash the dishes and this seemed to please him. At the end he spoke again, "Young friend on the Way, let us take a short stroll on these mountain paths; strange and inspiring are nights in these hills and perhaps we can, after all, learn something about the spirit of our ancient patriarchs. Then off to sleep, for dawn comes early east of the ridge."

His telepathic understanding of my unspoken questions had ceased to amaze me (I recalled how my Teacher at White Cloud Monastery had often plumbed my depths with his serene gaze), and we soon set forth. How the stars glistened in the clear air over the hills! Jupiter was bright at midheaven and Venus in the West, shining like a beacon in the darkening sky. He began to hum a tune; he obviously loved nocturnal perambulations on mountain paths. I too felt uplifted; the stars had never seemed so close and the perfect stillness of the mountain gave greater possibility of attunement to the celestial music and harmonies. For the first time I felt the inner movement of the heavens, the rhythmical processions, ever changing, yet eternal. He too seemed rapt, gazing upwards with hands clasped behind him. Presently he spoke. "Yes, dear friend, like you, I too was a scholar for many years. I read our ancient Classics—Confucius, Meng Zi, the Neo-Confucians, many Buddhist sutras, and of course our great old father Lao-Tze, the wisest, simplest, and most subtle. For many years I wandered the length and breath of this land with my Tao-friend Purple Gold, and it was he who at last convinced me that true wisdom was not to be found in books and teachings—though, as you can see, I have yet to wean myself entirely from this 'chaff of the ancients'—but in Nature herself. Then I came here and the previous dweller in this place transmitted to me the true teaching."

He paused a while and continued scanning the heavens. Not even a breeze rustled the trees below the path.

"Shall I give you the True Transmission you have been awaiting for so long? I know you will be very disappointed, because it is nothing special at all. First I had better give you some weightier stuff, so you will not feel you have made this long journey in vain. Does not the Earth follow the Way of Heaven? Without the Four Seasons and the celestial bodies—sun, moon, and planets—how could life and breath flourish here? Does not the sun warm us and beget all life? Do not the timely rains come to nourish the bosom of earth, so she can bring all things to birth?

"Were it not for Heaven, Earth could not produce, for warmth, moisture, the ocean tides, the flow of sap in trees, the probing of roots into the soil—all follow the movements of sun and planets. So Earth must pattern itself after Heaven, and Man, to become healthy, must likewise model himself after celestial rhythms; such is the origin or, more precisely, one of the origins, of our Taoist movement systems. Taiji and Ba Gua follow the movements of Heaven; Xing I follows more the ways of Earth and there are countless minor schools. As for Taiji, do not the slow stately movements express the grandeur of the heavenly procession itself? Gazing into the starry sky, the ancient founders and patriarchs saw that there was regularity, a constancy of movement, precise cycles of recurrence and flow. Also, are not the motions of sun, moon, stars, and planets smooth, without drastic breaks or leaps, steady and enduring? Moreover, all their movements appear circular, as the heavenly bodies themselves are circular. And there is the perpetual alternation of light and dark, warm and cold, as the sun processes through the four seasons, through each day and night, and as the moon alternately waxes and wanes.

"Our forerunners of olden times began to create arts of exercise-meditation-enjoyment, self-defense that embodied regular movements, circular in form, progressing in stately rhythm, alternating with the flow of Yin and Yang. When we move this way morning and evening, we come to sense in ourselves the steadiness of celestial rhythms, the grace and repose that comes from rounded movements, repeating themselves with subtle variations. Our character comes to be rounded, avoiding extreme positions, because we know that everything changes. We begin to enjoy a deep rapport with the course of the seasons, with the phases of the moon, for we feel in our small bodies an inner movement akin to the grander gestures of the heavens."

He fell silent for a long time and sat, leaning against a large boulder that bordered the path. Though night was deep, the sky was marvelously luminous, stars incredibly clear. I thought of the strange light I had seen the previous evening in the hill gap and glanced back towards the hut. No light—all was deep in the silence of ink blue sky. I thought of asking him about this, but the question seemed facetious. Hollow Valley had already spoken at some length, which I had not expected, and I didn't wish to impose on his silences. I thought of a passage from the Great Commentary to the *I Ching*:

> *Gazing up (we use it) to contemplate the celestial patterns; looking down, we examine the earthly markings, and thus come to know the causes of the dark (hidden) and the light (manifest)... it encompasses the transformations of Heaven and Earth, omitting nothing...(using it) we can penetrate the Tao of day and night, and understand it...The Sages (used it) to observe the movements of all under Heaven and contemplate their meetings and interpenetrations, coursing ever onwards in accordance with their own intrinsic principles.*

[From the *"Great Commentary"* on the *I Ching*—Author's translation.]

I felt Hollow Valley looking in my direction. "Let us return and sleep now; sleep is very close to Tao. The *I* is indeed a great teacher and I continue to study it daily, but truer teachers still are found overhead and underfoot." We returned in silence and I fell into a deep sleep immediately.

I awoke to find a cup of freshly brewed tea on a table near the bed, its fragrance still alive and the cup warm. My host was nowhere in sight. Dressing quickly, I entered the kitchen. There was a newly made pot of cooked rice and some soup, golden soup made from a kind of dried gourd and fresh roots. Delicious! I ate gratefully, my appetite very sharp from yesterday's long walk and our nightly trek up the mountain path. Though the morning was still very young, my host seemed to have already left to attend to some errand or perhaps simply stroll along the hillside. I washed the dishes and tidied the kitchen, a small task because everything was already perfectly ordered. I explored the hut and found no other sleeping quarters; evidently Hollow Valley had given me his "bedroom." I surmised he was off culling herbs somewhere, finding them with dew still fresh on their leaves. (Some of the very young and tender shoots would be at their best this early in the season.)

The bracing air of morning proved irresistible; I decided to walk the ridge in the daylight, admire the view, perhaps find some herbs to take back to the hut and surprise my host, though I was quite sure he knew the whereabouts of any substantial stand of plants. In about a quarter of an hour Hollow Valley was visible, bending close to the earth in a grove to the north of the path. As I approached, I could see several very mature ginseng plants. My host raised his hand, as if to caution me not to come closer. Then he walked over, took my arm, and we returned to the path. "Dear guest, these old roots and leaves are most precious indeed. They were tended by my predecessor here and were first planted many, many years ago. They most fully combine heavenly and earthly forces, drawing mysterious energies from sky and soil, as does the body of man himself, hence their name. And, since they are used only for the most precious medicine, we approach them but rarely, and my teacher here asked that on one go near them but dwellers on this hillside. Come, let us stroll. You will stay here yet a few hours, then I will be off on a short journey of several days' duration, and I doubt very much that we will meet again."

We walked off the path into a sort of gently sloping ravine. A rock wall was visible at the end, from which a clear spring bubbled merrily in the morning sun. Hollow Valley took two wooden buckets and a long bamboo pole from a small shed built around a turn in the rocky outcropping. When the buckets were filled he arranged the pole, shouldered it with one swift movement, and set off back to the path. He seemed not too disposed to conversation, so we proceeded in silence. The birdsong was exceptionally happy on this fine morning of spring and from time to time my host would respond in perfect melody. He seemed to be enjoying himself immensely, not at all burdened with the two heavy buckets, sniffing the air and laughing....

When we returned to the hut, he busied himself about the garden for a while, gently moistening and loosening the earth around the green sprouts. After some time had passed, and he seemed satisfied with his work, he sat down under a gnarled old pine and beckoned.

"Last evening we spoke of the heavens and Heaven is indeed the Grand Progenitor. But one who practices Tao will not neglect the patterns of Earth. Is she not the mother of all? We must come to understand her elusive inner movements, the subtle flow of life energy that courses through her veins, the patterns of movement in rock, tree, stream, and cloud. How rich our life becomes when we can feel in ourselves the soaring energy of spring clouds, the lilting motion of streams fed by late winter's melting snows, the resilient dance of a willow caressed by summer breezes. And what of the animals here? The ancient followers of the Way studied their habits and movements most carefully and modified them just enough so that we humans too could feel the strength of a crouching tiger, the sinuous grace of a coiling snake, the sublime nobility of a white crane spreading its wings. And what about a golden cock standing upright to meet the dawn or a wild horse carelessly tossing its mane in the wide open plains? When you perform the movements of our old Taoist exercise forms, you must absorb into yourself the energy, grace, and power of these lively animals. You can become as quick and nimble as a swallow skimming the water, as majestic as a great phoenix spreading wings. Feel the spirit, the joy in life of these fellow creatures, all of them true devotees of the Way. And do not forget the deep veins and arteries of Earth herself, full of life-giving water and *qi*. Perhaps you would like to see this treatise written by a scholar of old." He handed me a small scroll and went into the hut. I unrolled it and read,

In the regions below the Earth are varying layers of soil and rock and flowing watercourses. These layers rest upon thousands of (types of) qi conduits, arrayed in myriad branches, veins, and openings. The firm and yielding flow back and forth, in ceaseless transformations. Refined and subtle, the veins interpenetrate like an axle rotating in the depths with close connections all around. There appears to be a bellows at work. This wondrous network extends out and joins together every part of the Earth's roots. They are neither metal, nor stone, nor earth, nor water—
Thousands and ten-thousands of horizontal and vertical veins

are like a warp and weft, weaving together in mutual embrace. The millions of miles of earth seem to hang and float on a huge ocean. Taking into account land and sea as part of Earth the veins connect with each other in a mysterious way, while the nature of the veins and the colors, tastes, and sounds, both of the earth, the waters, and the rocks, differ from place to place. In similar manner, animals, birds, herbs, trees, and all natural products differ in form and nature in various places.

If the qi of Earth can penetrate these veins, then the water and earth above will be fragrant and fertile...and all men and things will be pure and wise...But if the Earth's qi is obstructed, the water and soil and natural products will be bitter, cold, and withered...and men and things will be evil and dull.

The body of Earth resembles a human being. Around and below the watery abdominal organs, there is much heat; if it were not so, people could not digest their food or do work. Likewise, the Earth is extremely hot below the watery regions; if it were not so, how could it evaporate all the waters or disperse the accumulated yin qi? Most people, unable to perceive the meridians and channels, arrayed in order in the human body, think it is only a lump of solid flesh.

In similar manner, unable to perceive the veins and channels arrayed under the ground, they think the Earth is only a homogeneous mass. They are not aware that Heaven, Earth, humans and natural things all have their patterns and principles. Even a wisp of smoke, a broken bit of ice, a fragment of a wall, or an old tile has its patterns and principles. (So) how can anyone say that the Earth does not have its patterns and principles?

[Cheng Se-Xiao
Late Sung Period
Author's translation]

I sat for a short while until a melodious bell sounded from within the little house. Entering, I found Hollow Valley seated at the table, a small traveling bundle by his side. "Let us partake of another frugal meal in silence, dear friend, before I journey north. I hope you have found the meager fare acceptable. Though tasteless, it provides sustenance for body and mind. You'll find few 'tasty dishes here to make a passing stranger pause.'" We exchanged a brief smile at this allusion, and began to eat. The food tasted marvelous: flavors smoothly blended; textures and colors in perfect harmony: A hearty broth of rice and barley, with many vegetables of varying colors and shapes. I wondered whether he would remember his promise to reveal the "True Transmission." Or had it been transmitted already through his observations and our walks? I decided to ask just before he departed; it seemed most unlikely I would come that way again and he seemed quite convinced that we would not have another meeting. Strange to say, most of the questions and doubts that had propelled me onto this journey, begun several weeks before, had now dissolved, so I did not feel desperate about the "True Transmission." Still, I resolved to probe him a bit if it proved necessary.

After the meal we sipped some light golden wine that bore an aroma of flowers and herbs and he filled my flask from an oddly shaped earthenware pitcher. "The true Elixir of Immortality," he beamed, "distilled from herbs and plants that grow on these hillsides. Should need arise, I could easily live on this wine and a small amount of rice for weeks on end, as I have often done through the winters here. You will find that it gives you good strength for your further travels. Let us go now. Though this is my home of homes, I often wander east and west. It is by good fortune that we were able to meet."

He picked up his bundle and headed for the door; I followed, most reluctant to part from him. Since the previous evening I had felt a deep and enduring contentment, as one sometimes feels with a very old friend whose mere presence confers joy and peace of mind. I hoped he would stay longer. He went out and sat down in the garden on a stone that I noticed was carved in an octagonal shape with the Trigrams on each face and a Taiji diagram on top. "My favorite sitting stone: Here I watch my plants grow, observe the seasons passing, spend many hours enjoying moonlight and the starry fires in the deep vault of space. Are you still awaiting the True Transmission? You do appear much calmer than yesterday; perhaps you no longer need it."

I was about to reply when he went on, "Dear Jin-An, it seems I'd better pass it on to you, else you may depart from here feeling as though you had missed something of importance. But in truth we have dealt with all the important matters already. In a sense the True Transmission is the least important, for there is really <u>nothing</u> to transmit. It is just this — *the secret of emptiness.* Can you be always empty and receptive? 'Blank as a piece of uncarved wood, yet receptive as a hollow in the hills?' Did not our Old Master say, 'Abiding in Creative Emptiness, one can contemplate the mysterious wonder of things...?' This is the true source of Tao. When no stray thought moves, the Tao can flow through you, its movement unimpeded. Thus the ancient practitioners of the Way abandoned their sagely wisdom to become still and empty like a hollow valley. In this way they were able to unite with the pulsing energies of everything around them and to enter freely into the creative life of Tao itself. No, the knowledge of Tao does not depend on books, or letters, university professors, priests or hierophants, though all of these have their rightful role to play. *Simply search your own mind for the secret of creative emptiness, letting no prejudicial thought enter your breast. Also, in every encounter of daily life treat all things around you with thoughtfulness, consideration, and care for all creatures are the vessels of Tao and through them Tao will manifest itself to you.* And now farewell, I must be off. We may meet again in a faraway place and time; transformation and change are ever the movement of the Way. Perhaps I'll be a twisted old tree and you a weary wayfarer, or you might become herbal wine and I a thirsty traveler; Or you an autumn cicada and I the evening breeze; Or I a falling snowflake and you a mountain stone. Nothing gets lost, dear friend, everything changes."

He slung the bundle over his shoulder and bowed low. I bowed to the ground and our eyes met for the last time. He strode up the hillside and I returned to the world of men.

Musings On a Golden Day
(or, the True meaning of Immortality)

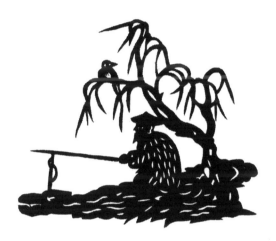

With thanks to Gracie for a day
on Cape Cod, and to Spring Dawn
for her shining spirit...

Musings on a Golden Day

Since the beginning of our acquaintance Peter Stuart had always seemed enigmatic and inscrutable, despite his appearance of ease and joviality. I first met him many years ago while we were fellow scholars in Beijing, immersing ourselves in the lore of the grand old Middle Kingdom before the Revolution. In those days he had devoted himself mainly to the literary arts and was a surpassing calligrapher, his secondary love landscape painting. Thus, it was not unusual to find him in places particularly beautiful, quietly seated and contemplating. And that was how we met.

One day near Qing Ming, that great spring festival 105 days after Winter Solstice, when families usher in the vernal clime by going into the countryside, sweeping their ancestral graves, drinking wine and picnicking, I was out in the suburbs strolling along, enchanted by the burgeoning beauties of the flatlands and gentle hills. When I arrived at the Court of Five Brilliances, a small Taoist temple that was often my haunt at holiday time, I noticed a foreigner sitting alone in the courtyard observing the swaying branches. Though he was clothed in antique garb his shock of reddish blond hair made it impossible to mistake him for a direct descendant of the Yellow Emperor. We shared a few words and I learned he was a devotee of Taoist lore; his knowledge of spoken and archaic Chinese well nigh flawless. He also seemed gifted in the meditative arts; though he mentioned nothing about this, his eyes emitted the sparkling glow touched with mellow good humor that bespeaks one well advanced in cultivating the Way.

Though we did not prolong our conversation at that time, in the intervening years we had become fast friends and often made pilgrimages together into the mountain districts seeking special beauty spots and historical sites.

Now, years later, walking along Marlborough Street, Boston, on a crystalline autumn afternoon, I wondered at the import of his urgent message that had reached me a few days before. It said only that he wanted to meet me as soon as possible, that he had a special missive for me that he had just received from abroad. We agreed to meet in the Public Garden on nine-nine day, the ninth day of ninth lunar month, dedicated to the North Star Deity, patron of Taoist internal martial arts. But what a day! Golden leaves cascading down everywhere, contrasting delicately with the soft red patina of Back Bay brick. Young people sauntering along Beacon St., playing out the eternal rounds of college life in the autumn, scenes I remembered so well. The bracing air of fall football afternoons, fresh romances, homecomings, parties....

Beacon and Arlington—I crossed the street and entered the Garden, not quite sure where I would meet my old comrade. It wasn't long before I spotted him sitting near one of the old stone lanterns adjacent to the bridge and lagoon. As I approached from the rear, I could see he was wearing an old slightly rumpled grayish suit, but a bright green beret at a rakish angle adorned his mass of flaming hair, giving him a lithe and youthful appearance. I was quite certain he did not notice me draw near, but as I came up he turned and rose, graciously saluting me with the traditional Taoist bow. He then sat down again and motioned me to be seated next to him. With Peter I had long ago come to expect extended periods of silence.

He felt the need to say little, but being with him was a communication in itself. He was preternaturally sensitive to any change in his surroundings and delighted in observing subtle wonders that would elude most other people. By sitting near him and "tuning in," I was often able to bring mental chatter to a halt and become acutely aware of colors and sounds, gestures and motions. Often the aggregate of it all would blend into a marvelous sound-color-dance and few places were better for this than the Public Garden on an October afternoon. He seemed delighted in the patterns of movement woven by sailing Frisbees, dogs, women pushing carriages, frolicking children, strolling lovers.

His attention was particularly arrested by one beautiful little girl who looked not more than three years old. Sun-haired and rosy cheeked, wearing a pink cotton frock, she was ambling along the periphery of the lagoon, gazing deeply into the murky water. Strange to say, no parent was near; she walked on for a long time, occasionally chuckling to herself and looking up with a delighted expression. Now and then she would skip a few steps, eyes dancing and smiling; then resume her slow perambulation of the lagoon. I became more and more puzzled, but Peter just watched, his face a mixture of benevolence and amusement. He seemed utterly unconcerned about any danger to the girl, but I was becoming more and more alarmed. He placed his palm gently on my arm, "What are you fretting about?" he asked, "Everything's under control. See her mother over there, sitting on the bench across the water? She seems to be reading to her blind son, but she is totally aware of every movement made by her small daughter over here. You may doubt this, but she also knows, without understanding how, that I would speedily rescue her daughter, should anything untoward happen. But it won't; her <u>awareness</u> is protecting the child, and moreover the child is a special one safeguarded by benevolent powers. Why this is so, I can't say."

We sat a few more moments and I became progressively calmer; being with Peter for a while, one couldn't help but feel at peace, that everything was evolving as it should, and that "Tao was taking care of everything."—one of his favorite expressions. "Well, I do have something special for you, and sunset is a good time to recall old friends. Shall we go?" I nodded and we set off across Beacon Street to his apartment overlooking the Charles Esplanade. A perfect time for being there! Clouds just beginning to be tinged with golden-rose and the water a deep blue-gray, cold under the crisp sky.

I always felt happy and at ease in Peter's apartment. Though the furnishings were by no means opulent, each piece had been selected with an impeccable aesthetic sense and preserved with loving care. There was a feeling of airiness and space in his large studio, but the elegant arrangement of line and color gave the place a most agreeable warmth and coziness. We settled ourselves comfortably—he on the velvet maroon sofa near the fireplace and I at a small beautiful carved teak tea table near the window from which I could see the Longfellow and Harvard bridges and the boats on the river, their sails afire in the waning sunlight, returning to the boathouses.

He lit a couple of small lamps and then reached for his favorite tobacco can and pipe. "You know I can't stand tea, but please help yourself to whatever your taste fancies. There is some passably good leaf here and if you don't mind the fragrance of my pipe, we can chat a bit of old times and places." I discovered a small canister of Wild Mountain tea (*ye shan cha*) in the pantry and heated some water. Soon there was an ambrosial infusion from the old square Ming Dynasty teapot I remembered so well from our many meetings and talks in China. "Ah ha, you found it, as I thought you would! Then do take it, for it is yours. I always like to have some decent tea around for my old friends and the *ye shan cha* is for you." I thanked him warmly. Wild Mountain is one of the rarest types, the one Chinese prize most dearly, and never available outside the country. I had not enjoyed any for a number of years and my nose and palate were aglow with anticipation at the very thought of tasting this precious elixir once again.

Peter's dislike of tea was completely incomprehensible to me, as it was to his Chinese friends and colleagues, but we soon became accustomed to his abstention and to his great enjoyment of the pipe, which he would discreetly puff at a distance if the tea we were sipping was especially prized for its fragrance. This and his total aversion to *keqi hua* (Chinese mannered polite conversation) were the only aspects of his character that seemed out of keeping with his great erudition in and love of things Chinese, but I believed they actually endeared him in some special way to his Chinese hosts.

Once I was settled with my tea and he was cozy with a well-drawing pipe, he began, "A few days ago I received a package from a Mr. Meng, whom I believe you may remember. He was a disciple of the Taoist Purple-Gold for quite a long time, and served his Master almost continuously for the last five years of his life. According to the stories, he was the son of a famous general and his mother's family had been traditional physicians for some six generations. He grew up interested in the martial arts and medicine, trained at several temples, then entered official life. After his father's death he resigned his post and devoted all his time to practicing medicine, eventually forming a lucrative practice in Shanghai. He had a palatial home, many concubines, several country estates, and a large business trading in medicinal herbs. Some time in his late fifties, he is said to have met Purple-Gold on one of his journeys to the Shandong Peninsula. At that time Purple-Gold was still vigorous, though rich in years, and was himself traveling to Mr. Hua for a while, then returning northeast.

"The accounts say that Meng then sold all his goods and businesses, saw to the provision of his wife and family (he had three grown sons at the time), and traveled to Shandong, where he begged to be admitted to personal discipleship with Purple-Gold. I don't know whether Purple-Gold accepted this; he was loathe to play the master role in any sense, but he did allow Mr. Meng to remain with him during the last five years of his life, together with a small group of others who had taken him as their teacher. But I had better let our mysterious Mr. Meng speak for himself..."

He opened a lacquered trunk that I remembered from China and withdrew a packet of papers, which he handed to me. "To you from Mr. Meng.... How he discovered my present address I have no idea, but a letter came a few days ago saying that I must find you and give you the enclosed letters. You are most welcome to stay here and read them if you wish; you know I won't consider it impolite if you peruse them at leisure. I need to write a few characters anyway; even one day without practice and my wrist begins losing suppleness; four or five days off and my brush, which one old master said should be soft as a willow wand waving in the wind, starts to feel like a creaky old doorpost. I prefer the willow wand..." As Peter began preparing his paper and ink, I opened the packet.

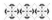

To Jin-An:

Esteemed Sir, enclosed please find a letter from the Purple-Gold Taoist. Though I believe the two of you met but once, he seemed to have a special fondness for you and during the last few days of his life spoke of his chance meeting with you on several occasions. He evidently felt some sort of deep karmic connection with you and on the last day of his sojourn in this realm, he handed me the enclosed parcel, asking that I find you wherever you might be—he was certain that I <u>would</u> eventually find you—and deliver this to you. I, an insignificant dreamer on the Path, had the good fortune to be Purple-Gold's follower for more than five years. Since we are, in a sense, brother disciples, I will relate to you the events during his last few days.

At the time of which I write Purple-Gold was well advanced in years, though he would tell no one his exact age. His hair, still long and drawn into a bun on top of his head, was shining white, gracefully complementing his strong ruddy face. In fact, right up to his death he was the very picture of health and few of us younger men could keep up with him on his treks through the mountains. Five days before his Transmutation (though none of us had the slightest inkling as to his departure from this world), he called together the small band of disciples which had gathered around his retreat on the Shandong Peninsula, and told us that this would be a special time for him and for us and that we should keep a quiet mind and observe everything carefully.

Each morning we rose three hours before dawn and the meditations were especially long and deep; the diurnal activities were much the same as usual, but Purple-Gold seemed strangely luminous during those days. His good humor was superb; he would go down to the village for several hours each day to play with the youngsters, and at night there were again long meditations by candlelight, followed by many ancient chants. We weren't sure why he seemed to be celebrating so, thinking perhaps it was to commemorate some special event in his distant past. Yet none of us could remember a similar period during the time we had known him.

After about three days, we began to realize what was happening, though none of us would speak of it aloud. Indeed, there seemed nothing ominous about it; slowly the consciousness that he was shortly to return to the True Home began to dawn in us. A certain worldly sadness took hold, surely, but the overall feeling was almost elated. It was impossible to be sad or gloomy around this old man.

On the fifth day he called us to his hut for a special ceremony at midnight. We lit the finest incense, drank tea, and held a special session of chanting to the Three Pure Ones, Lao, and Chuang. Then we sat rapt in meditation until sunrise, when Purple-Gold descended the steep path to the sea-edge and lightly bathed. Rinsing himself with some fresh water, which he must have set nearby the night before, he attired himself in his finest garments, white trousers and a deep blue traveling robe with immense butterfly sleeves embroidered in patters of dragon and phoenix, which he had worn on his pilgrimages to the Sacred Mountains. During breakfast at which he did not eat, he addressed us as follows,

"Dear companions on the Path! Today is a day of special journey for me and I am happy to enjoy this time with you, as I have been glad to share these several years. I have always been a wanderer, a traveler, a pilgrim along the endless Way and I thank you from my heart for your company on some of my recent journeys. It seems our next travels together will take place when we have all reunited in the cloud palaces of the Immortals, borne there, perhaps, on the backs of white cranes sporting and dancing in the sunlight. As to 'cultivating Tao,' be assured that no pursuit is quite so fruitless. Tao cannot be cultivated, for it interfuses everything we see, hear, do, and touch; our very life breath <u>is</u> the Way itself. Can you cultivate this? It would not be amiss, however, if you sought diligently for the unblemished clarity of your deepest inner spirit, for there Tao will come alive for you, and all else besides."

After that he retired to his hut for a while and busied himself writing a long letter, which I now understand is the one contained in this package for you. Around noontime he summoned us together and walked several miles down the road to one of his favorite minor pilgrimage spots, a red and azure lacquered pavilion overlooking the sea. The day was lightsome and the ocean blue glowed deep under the autumnal sun; the bronze hue of the season touched and burnished the wooded hillsides; here and there brilliant red or gold patches highlighted the more subdued groves and copses. We halted and he remained silent for a while, contemplating the gently lapping waves; the tide was in and the water swelled to the very edge of the cliff below, yet there was no wind and the seas were beautifully calm.

He seated himself and began,

"Centuries ago and even up to our own time, emperors, Taoist masters, alchemist, poets, and seekers after marvels have come to these coasts and gazed across these very waters. It is said that the Isles of the Blest lie beyond in the Eastern Seas. As you are aware, many persons tried to discover these isles, but few returned and those who did always came back with only stories of apparitions and mirages to tell.

"Truly, the Immortals are elusive and not easily approached by would-be seekers of endless life. And yet—what a tragic mistake these pilgrims made! For all they needed to know about Immortality was right here beneath their eyes and feet all the while.

"Some of you, the newer disciples in particular, still occasionally question me about the meaning of Immortality. Or ask about my teachers and lineage. Fruitless queries! However, since you have befriended me, taken part in my life and shared my daily practice for many years, I have decided to introduce you to my teachers."

A stir of anticipation passed through the group and some of the younger apprentices looked up, as if expecting to behold the approach of some magnificent figure, such as Fu Xi or the Jade Emperor. But we older disciples smiled quietly; we had finally understood.

"Yes, followers of the Way with me, allow me the honor of introducing you to my greatest teacher, Eastern Ocean, and his inseparable companions, Tai Yang and Tai Yin. How they ebb and flow, roar and purl, tumble and dance together endlessly! The golden and silver orbs ever arising out of and returning to the dark and heaving bosom of the waters. They go about their appointed rounds ceaselessly, yet never in haste and never complaining. They bring moisture, light, warmth, food, and solace to countless beings, yet never claim lordship. The Ocean, for all its immensity, is ever obedient to the Queen of Night, and shapes its tides accordingly; Tai Yin herself, revolving faithfully from millennium to millennium, keeping the time for our planting, celebrations, births, and death, is herself content to radiate the glow of the Sun.

"And Tai Yang—its light comes from the mysterious darkness of Tao itself, which is faster and more dynamic than any light. 'Dark and mysterious—and yet more dark and mysterious—the gateway to all wonders.' The points of light from all distant stars and galaxies arise out of the infinite creative emptiness of Tao, which we perceive as 'darkness'. But that is only so because most people lack sufficient speed to perceive that the dusky vaults of space are brilliant with endlessly coursing patterns of liquid gold. When these slow down and congeal, they begin to form galaxies and heavenly bodies, which then become perceptible to the vision of men.

"In my younger days I studied all manner of sacred books, especially the *Book of Change* and Lao Tze, not to mention many of Lord Buddha's sutras and numerous treatises on alchemy, meditation, and suchlike. But words are endless and bring one no closer to the Way. Finally I realized that my Teachers had never been apart from me. Each day I rose to salute the dawning Sun as my dear brother, greeted the Moon as sister, gazed into the silent immensity of the night until the heavens began to glisten with pathways of golden liquid. I watched the currents of mountain mists and observed the interplay of hills and marshes, lakes and meadows. And when I was not traveling inland, I always returned to Eastern Ocean, my teacher and friend.

"I needn't burden you with more words; I am no longer a youth and find no delight in glib talk. But if you would follow my Teachers, first empty your own minds; then watch and merge into the lights of Sun and Moon and the motions of Wind and Wave. Understand the faith and humbleness of these teachers on whom we rely for our very life and who serve us endlessly. Know the true activity and meaning of Yang, Yin, and the bottom of the Sea. Once you accomplish this, you will have no more questions about Immortality."

He stood gazing into the waters a long time, then said he wanted to return home and greet the setting sun. We climbed slowly back up the cliffside path. Upon reaching home, he went in for a short time and appeared to be arranging his belongings. The he emerged and asked us on no account to disturb him for the next several hours.

He had brought a small cushion and seated himself atop a rock, gazing out to sea in the direction of the setting sun. By now none of us had any doubt as to the meaning of his actions, and we retired to a nearby house to watch and wait. Stillness prevailed; none of us was in the least disposed to carry on conversation. As the molten sun extinguished itself in the gray-green sea, we seemed to hear the strains of an ancient melody coming from Purple-Gold's sitting rock. Then all was silent.

As evening's chill pervaded the air, we began to wonder about the Master. None of us wanted to disturb him, but we were becoming concerned. As I was the eldest disciple, they prevailed on me to go and see what was happening. I approached the Master quietly, walked around him and stopped. Through the dimming light I could see his face glowing and still rosy, and he was sitting very erect with just the hint of a smile curling his lips. He seemed to be meditating still, so I went back to the others.

Midnight came with no change. Purple-Gold remained erect facing the darkened waters. This time I went up and gently touched his cheek; it was still warm, though he did not seem to be breathing. Unsure what to do, we formed a semi-circle around him and gradually entered meditation until just before the dawn. As the gentle sunlight of early morning touched our backs, I again approached the Master, to find that his face was as radiant as it had been last night and his skin still emitted warmth, though it was obvious his breath had long ceased. We discussed what to do and thought it unseemly to leave him on his rock any longer; we brought him into his hut and seated him facing west on his usual meditation spot. Then we noticed that all his belongings had been neatly packaged and labeled. Each of us received some small gift—a statuette of Lao Tze for one, old books for another, a favorite wine cup for another, and there were some herbal medicines of great value for his friends in the village. He had also made some amulets, carved with sportive animal figures for several of his favorite children, who were his frequent visitors. And there was the letter for Jin-An, which you now hold in your hands.

Since the passing of Purple-Gold most of us have dispersed, but we meet from time to time. He did not want to start any organization or formal temple. One of us, however, remains living in his hut at his request to entertain any passing traveler who might need shelter in that area.

"During my wandering days I often regretted not being able to afford my friends and guests gracious hospitality, having no place to shelter or entertain them. Now that I have returned to the Source, my *po* and *hun* will occasionally reunite to enjoy the fragrant essences of fine wine or tea with friends who come to visit me...ha ha."

His body remained warm for three days, then gradually cooled, though he remained sitting all the while. At sunset the fourth day we committed his body, still clothed in antique traveling robe, to the earth on a hilltop close to his Teachers. At this time one of our number, Wind Dragon, still tends the Master's house and small garden, and offers shelter to passing travelers. He is also a superb flute player, hence his name.

I take the liberty of enclosing a few of his poems, which we found in the hut. He is said to have befriended a wandering Japanese monk many years ago and the poems, I think you'll agree, show much influence of Japanese style, their metrical structure not based on our ancient ways. Perhaps we will meet when the affinities are right; I greet you as a friend on the Path and brother disciple.

wishing you peace of heart
and long life

Meng

Poems by Purple-Gold

The midnight mockingbird has long been silent,
Even the cat is deep in dreams.
Only this hermit keeps on writing,
Meteors play tag in the vast open sky.

Wind-blown mists on a summer's evening
The world sleeps on
while daffodils toss their heads...

Sitting on a stone tomb under the swaying oaks,
I become aware of the meaning of Life and Death.
No big thing really —
The white clouds will tell us,
If only we listen

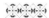

Cicadas sing to an October's dawn,
Oblivious to summer's passing.
A ripe thorn apple
drops on the white dew.

Three hawks wheeling high,
dawn moon falls
into an empty sky.

Letter from Purple Gold to Jin-An
Musings on a Golden Day

To Tao-friend Jin-An, greetings from afar...

Jin-An, dear friend on the Way, many times since our chance meeting in a pavilion my thoughts have turned to you, an ancient wandering companion from many past lifetimes. Since today is a very special day for me, I send you this message, which will be my last during this cycle of time, for today I return to the source (from which I have never departed!). Meanwhile, let me bow in greeting to you and send you a few words on what we Taoists call "Immortality." What a silly thing to talk or write about! One could easily ask the trees, birds, or stones for their wisdom. Yet followers of the Way for countless generations have sought Immortality in its many forms, and I too was a seeker for many a long year, up to age sixty or thereabouts. But my wanderings over the last forty years have changed all that...

It is a day here I should like to share with you, could you but be here to join my small family of Tao friends. I sit in my small stone house, in which I have dwelt these past five courses of the Seasons. Below, the ocean sparkling silver-blue; nearby stalks of grain ripen in the golden warmth of Long Summer and toss their heads in sprightly dance to every passing breeze. Often deer venture into the pine grove beyond the stream and we have become good friends; looking deeply into their eyes, I wonder and rejoice at their wise and shining spirit. I have many friends here—the grand blue sky, winter winds and summer clouds, morning mists and evening chill; the very world is a magnificent dance.

Though my wandering heart is still much with me, these several years I have watched here, so close to earth and sea; Heaven and Earth provide all my needs and there is much time to ripen in the Way. Few people know the earthly age of this traveler, but I have passed my 104th journey around the yearly sun seven days ago and that very evening as I reclined with incense and candlelight, gazing out my window beyond the dusk into the merging of water and sky, one of the ancient Patriarchs appeared and gave me call, so I knew I should soon be returning to the Mother. Now here I am, an old man of white hair and beard, so content with my tea, cakes brought to me by village children, the warmth of the sun and splashing of waves, and the companionship of my younger friends.

Shall I speak of Immortality? From the time of the Yellow Emperor we Taoists have been practicing all sorts of methods to attain this elusive and chimerical state. No doubt some have achieved it, but it is usually not what common men understand by the word. We revere Lao and Chuang as great teachers on the Way, yet it is not recorded that either engaged in *xian* practice. And of the many who have engaged in such practices, all but very few came to rest under the green hills, as is the fate of wayfarers from all times and paths. Other followers to Tao have eschewed all such paths, engaging instead in the joys of limpid conversation (*qing tan*), wine, poetry, and love. And I can assure you that these paths are truly ways to merge with the Way, less dangerous and arduous than *xian* practices. As for this recluse, dear friend, he has at one time or other gone down all of these paths. Brought up as the son of an Imperial Tutor, I was early exposed to the *Four Books* and *Five Classics.* But my inner penchant was always for the scriptures of Tao and I would read and meditate on these night and day, to my father's great displeasure. My greatest interest lay in the treatises on alchemy and Immortality; I became obsessed by the golden Elixir and questioned many of my Taoist friends about it. I began to secretly study meditation and internal energy techniques. My father was severely discomfited by my practices and was mollified only by my assiduous study of the Confucian classics; naturally he wanted me to become a high ranking official.

I passed the *jin-shih* (Imperial scholars') examination at age eighteen and continued my studies both formal (Confucian) and secret (Taoist). Six years later my father passed away and, after observing the three years' period of mourning, I established myself in a separate house and courtyard of my family mansion in the capital. Here I began Immortality practices in earnest. I had many close friends among the local Taoist elite at that time, so there was no lack of instruction. I observed special dietetic regimens, practiced strictly regulated breathing yogas, meditated for many hours each morning and evening, as well as practicing several martial arts and *qigong* systems. My body became strong and light; my health was superb and my senses clear. The world became so bright to me! The leaves on the trees shone radiant; the scent of each flower and herb seemed to penetrate my very being. During those years I also enjoyed painting and calligraphy, spent many hours ambling in the hills enjoying the splendors of nature with my friends. How to describe the intoxication of walking mountain paths to greet the full moon as she emerged from glowing shrouds of mist? Or the cool mornings of early spring when we would trip gaily along rushing streams while all the world came awake and alive! I was also privileged in a special way in those younger days. For several years I practiced the yogas of Green Dragon/White Tiger, hoping in this way to find entry to the world of the Immortals. The incandescent glow and ecstasy of the perfect meeting of Yin and Yang surpassed all description. Yet, as time went on, I began to wonder...

Now, midway through my fourth cycle of twelve years, I began to perceive the futility of all my earlier practices. I was still unmarried, a source of extreme disappointment to my mother and uncle. Several times they had come close to arranging a betrothal for me, yet each time I was able to elude them. Moreover, I had by now acquired the reputation of being somewhat eccentric, and since I had no official post, it was very difficult to find suitable young ladies of good family. I was still well known from previous years for my scholarly attainments, so there was no lack of opportunity to tutor aspiring candidates for the Imperial Examinations; in this way my material needs were adequately met. I enjoyed a most gracious and elegant life in the great Northern Capital. But my quest for Immortality was beginning to prove burdensome.

Finally, after traversing these many paths, tasting of their joys and sorrows, their follies and moments of sublime inspiration, I left it all and began the life of a voyager among clouds and streams around age forty. And it was not until several decades later, as I sat near the sea one day on a stone tomb watching the blue clouds glide overhead that it all became clear to me.

We cannot practice, nor gain Immortality, for we are already Immortal! All that we can and must do is refine the body (hence the value of Taoist yogas, martial arts, and inner purifications) and plumb the depth of our clear spirit until we realize in our very bones that we and Tao are one. By treating each thing around us with affection and care, taking as little from Nature as necessity dictates, we find that benign Nature mysteriously protects us in each circumstance. Unsuspected energies and illuminations become available to us;

illness is non-existent or very rare; friends on the Path appear in greater and greater number. As time ripens, we start to understand the song of birds and breezes; Nature herself is pleased to instruct, protect, and guide us at all times.

Dear friend, the practice of "Immortality" is not to gain any sort of special powers of our own, but to make ourselves worthy of the benevolent protection of Tao itself. As we become ever more aware of the subtle flux of life energy and the movement of Tao, our hearts open to gladness and we understand the Creative Spirit with radiant clarity. Fellow beings find joy in our presence and have no <u>will</u> to harm us. This is the highest level of inner martial arts, the true way of peace. In the end we become a creature whom <u>Tao</u> is pleased to let live, rather than suffer harm. How then can we "die?" Without effort, we are part of the Always-So. This is the true meaning of Immortality practice and the furthest reach of the Taoist arts of "self-defense" and preservation of life.

Immortality is something which we must practice, yet cannot practice directly; the gift is given by Tao itself and can never be forced. Yet we can prepare ourselves to receive it, and then wait for our allotment, if it be our fate to be so favored. I now understand that all so-called *xian* practices are naught else but ways to prepare ourselves for a gift, or more precisely, to refine ourselves to appreciate and live most fully in the gifts we already possess.

Jin-An, you know of many methods, need I discuss them in detail? The schools of hygiene which concentrate the breath and *qi* internally; the schools of movement and martial practice; the schools of tranquil meditation; the schools of alchemy who concoct and decoct potions made from lead and cinnabar—alas, many would-be Immortals took the precepts of the ancient masters literally and returned to the Source sooner than they would have intended; the schools of rain and cloud; the schools of magic, divination, astrology, etc.—all are part of our Taoist tradition and all bear some claim to being part of the practice of Immortality. Yet perhaps, if erringly practiced, they miss the most important point of all. <u>We are the Tao already!</u> Why all this fuss?

Let yourself release completely, soar as freely as spring clouds in the blue sky; ebb and flow in utter trust as do the Four Seas, responding with no-mind to the promptings of sun and moon, planets and wind; let your life and gifts burgeon truthfully like the first plum blossoms bursting through the snows. Can you see? Everything is pulsing within and through the breath of Tao—you, I, and the Ten Thousand Things are "there" already, always have been and will be, though the changes of form are many. So do not waste too much time on methods and techniques, seek only the one empty sky of your own transparency and Tao will never be hidden from you. Tao is the light and shines always; our only task is to drop off that in us which obstructs the Light. For the radiant spring dawn is ever before us, have we but the eyes to see. May we meet again beyond time and distance.

Your friend on the Path,
Purple-Gold

A scent of tobacco smoke wafted across the room as I re-acclimated myself to the reality of sitting in an apartment overlooking Boston's Charles River Basin. Peter was still writing characters, pipe in mouth, as was his wont. He noticed I had finished reading.

"I have a feeling we may be hearing from Meng before too long. Right now you have that <u>distant</u> look, as though you're back in China. I won't disturb your inner feeling now, but autumn demands a suitable banquet and celebration. Can you return in three days?" We agreed and I left the letters for him to read. Coming out onto Beacon Street, I walked homeward into the darkening west.

[*xian*: is a term meaning "Immortal" composed of radical for "man" and "mountain." It came to be a generic term for varying schools of practice directed toward the attainment of extreme longevity, and in some cases, belief in a literal immortality of the body.]

A Butterfly's Dream

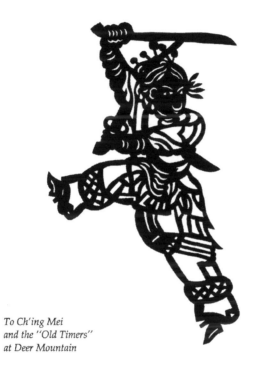

*To Ch'ing Mei
and the "Old Timers"
at Deer Mountain*

A Butterfly's Dream

The Zephyr pounded its way across the darkness of the cold Kansas prairie toward the rising sun. Heads propped on thin white AMTRAK pillows rocked in rhythm with the gentle sway of the coach. There were few awake; an old man who sat staring emptily out the window; a little boy who could not get comfortable and kept fidgeting and adjusting his body this way and that; two teenage girls chatting with youthful animation several rows ahead. I was in that gentle reverie of not quite awakeness, a time of numerous subconscious threads drawing themselves together and revealing hidden visions, dreams, and insights.

What a change of clime! The outdoors seemed bitter now; there was a chilling metallic sound to the clash of wheels and rails, and even from within the car there were probing fingers of icy breeze when the train stopped at rural stations. Just yesterday morning I had been in southern California, enjoying the smell of the ocean and the warm sun, with palm trees undulating in the on-shore breeze. But once through the desert and over the lower Rockies the reality of a hard Midwestern winter was becoming apparent. In some sense this long ride was good for me; the prolonged airlines strike provided an opportunity for a gradual journey home that would make way for the necessary psychological transition. I knew that my home would always be the soft mountains of western New England, yet for the past six years I had lived in southern California—an interesting change but one that I knew would not be permanent.

A perfect red solar disc ascended above the snow- covered plains, preceded by a wash of orange-rose and then by the golden streamers that betoken dawn in clear skies. The plain looked like a sea of glass; there must have been a warmer spell, possibly rain, and then a deep freeze. Smoke rising from farmhouses was almost vertical and had that white steamy look that shows frigid air. People were waking up all around me now, some off to the lounge for an early cup of coffee, others rubbing their eyes and adjusting for another day of travel. I took a few sips of tea and sat up straighter. In about twenty-five hours I would be home!

But it would not be an everyday homecoming. It would be something special. Ever since my last meeting with Peter Stuart in Boston, we had kept in frequent touch and though six years had elapsed since our last meeting, our friendship had deepened and seemed fresh as ever. He was, of course, ever unpredictable. And it was with no small surprise that I read his most recent letter, telling me that Mr. Meng had been living in north central Maine for almost a year with his eldest son and a small community of students. I was somewhat angry at his not having told me this sooner, but knowing Peter, he must have had his own reasons. In any event, the letter contained an invitation to visit Meng as soon as I came east.

How eagerly I looked forward to the journey's end! My stay in the West had been very hectic, professional activities taking up almost all of my time, and I had little chance to communicate at length with old friends. And I had heard nothing from Meng since receiving his letter from Purple-Gold. Still, in the deeper recesses of my consciousness I knew that I would one day meet Meng, though the precise time and situation were unclear to me. But I had never anticipated that he would now be living so close to my own home.

The remainder of the trip passed quickly enough. I had brought sufficient light food to sustain me during the passage and periodic exercise breaks on station platforms were enough to make me feel fit. East of Buffalo the land began to rise again, after the almost interminable flat whiteness of the plains. Soon the Hudson River valley appeared and then the winding route through the Berkshires of Western Massachusetts, particularly beautiful on this brilliant January morn. White steeples shown from behind pine clad hillsides and the small New England farmsteads were a cozy contrast to the extended acreage of the states to the west.

Finally! We pull into Boston's South Station at 9:24 AM. I am expecting Peter to meet me, but am greeted instead by a young man named Roger, who introduces himself as a student of Meng, and who will take Peter and me to Maine. Peter is now living in Winchester, a suburb to the northwest of the city and we are to meet him there and proceed to Meng's together. During our drive from South Station, Roger tells me about his history and connection with Meng. An electronics wizard ever since high school, he had studied computer science and worked in international finance and communications, but had then become increasingly restless and dissatisfied with this lifestyle. He was also growing seriously concerned about humanity's deteriorating relationship with Nature. During time off from his demanding schedule of career and family commitments he had worked with various "New Age" groups specializing in solar applications to heating, greenhouse gardening, and electrical power generation.

During this time he had turned to meditation, Zen Buddhist style, as a counterpoint to the tensions of his job and as an expression of his growing interest in a more integrated way of life. Nearing forty, he had also enrolled in a "kung-fu" class to keep in shape. Though robust and vigorous in his earlier years, he had begun to sense that his readiness to confront any problem or embark on new adventures was starting to wane. He felt weak and sluggish. His interest in "kung-fu" grew surprisingly. At first attending two one-hour classes weekly, he found himself after one year going for two hours every night and beginning to practice *qigong* and Taoist meditation in addition to his Forms and exercises. He had continued with his Buddhist practice, but felt more and more drawn to Taoism despite the frustration of finding no teachers who could aid his advance to deeper levels.

He had nonetheless acquired a strong healthy body after several years of practice and felt as well as he remembered feeling in his early twenties. He could now rise at dawn throughout the year to meditate and practice, and had begun to develop various abilities generally termed "psychic." In sparring sessions at the studio he found he could anticipate his partner's moves with ease, neutralizing attacks almost before they were initiated. And now he had an unerring sense of peoples' characters and future direction in life. Even so, his growing powers of prescience were unable to avert the untimely death of his wife in a plane crash. For about a year thereafter he remained shocked and depressed, knowing that his life's direction would no longer be the same. When he heard about Meng's arrival, he went to visit immediately. Both men liked each other at first sight, and within two months Roger and his two daughters had moved to Meng's community.

Peter was waiting on his front porch when we arrived, wrapped in a bright green muffler and jaunty cap, undaunted by the crisp weather. He was a dapper as ever and seemed not to have aged at all since our last meeting. Settling himself into the back seat, he lit his pipe and the stories began as soon as we were underway.

"Once Meng had discovered how to reach me, we kept in frequent contact and it became obvious that he was planning to come and live in the States. We discussed a number of places by mail until he decided on north central Maine, prompted by several revelatory dreams. He requested that I not tell you about this until he was fairly well established and we could all visit together. I myself have not yet been to his place, though we have met in Boston on various occasions." A small cloud of fragrant smoke wafted forward from the rear seat. "The California sun has done you good, my boy, you look healthier than when you left here. Still, I'm glad you are coming back. You were getting too immersed in busy-ness out there; and straying from the way of simplicity." He was right; it <u>was</u> time to return.

"Yes, training in Tao is a subtle matter," began Roger. "I know exactly what it is like to be overly involved with the 'dusty world.' For quite some time I lived the 'ideal' life—had a beautiful wife, lovely kids, and a well-paying profession. But when I did manage to give myself a little time to reflect and feel deeply what was going on inside, I always found this 'damn nothing' feeling. After a while I could hardly get out of bed in the morning—same old routines to look forward to. Sure, there were 'problems' and 'challenges', but nothing on any deeply satisfying level. No spirit in any of it. I was barely forty, yet would come home exhausted every night too tired to really enjoy my family, go to bed fatigued and wake up listless. Not a pretty picture. Much of that improved when I started Zen training and 'kung fu'. But the real turning point came when I lost my wife. She had been on a trip west to visit her parents and I was expecting her return flight to Boston in the late afternoon.

"Just after lunch I had a terrible feeling of urgency, of needing to be alone. I felt frightened and sick. Telling my secretary to cancel all my appointments for the next hour, I locked the door to my office and tried my best to enter a meditative state. Suddenly I <u>saw</u> my wife's face, fear-filled, yet calm, heard a loud whirring sound, cries and shouts, then a thunderous noise and dead silence. A moment later she appeared, radiant, calm and smiling. 'Don't worry,' she said, 'I am <u>beyond</u> now and all is at peace. Have no fear for me; I am in a world of light. Sorry I have to leave you and our daughters so soon, but please know our souls will always be joined, and I will await you and them in this shining place. Tell them I love them and all is well.'

Her image faded. I was in a state of utter shock and amazement, but somehow deeply at peace. I knew that my destiny had been forever altered and this was a sign directing me toward a new life.

"After affairs had been settled and my daughters had adjusted, I continued 'kung fu' classes. They were a sorely needed stabilizing influence in my life at that time. One of my classmates mentioned an elderly Chinese gentleman, a supposed 'Taiji master,' who was living in north central Maine. I found it hard to believe that a real 'Taiji master' would be living in so remote a location, and one day went to visit there with my classmate. As soon as I saw Meng, I knew that he was the teacher I had been waiting for and that from him I could learn the secrets of real internal practice. He told me a little of his plans and I was amazed by the breadth of his vision—a modern Taoist community in which the best aspects of modern science and Taoist knowledge would be conjoined. A place that would be immersed in the human-with-nature principles of Tao, yet responsive to today's world and its needs. He wanted to develop a community in which young people could be educated in self- reliance and martial arts, able to create their own way to health and inner integrity. He felt that many aspects of the traditional martial arts education, together with practical arts such as agriculture, herbal medicine, carpentry, and even electronics, could provide young people with a foundation for their own development of confidence and self-respect.

"He was also interested in creating a worldwide computer linked network of information on natural healing arts, herbs, agricultural methods, and nature-based use of modern technologies. I was stunned. Here was a 'traditional Chinese', educated in the old school, whose modernity of outlook rivaled that of the most 'far-out' New Agers! And I could be involved in something of importance to humanity while doing what I loved, learning deeper levels of martial arts, and living a healthy lifestyle. Within two months, we had moved to Meng's community at Purple Cloud Mountain. I felt as though I had been looking for this all my life.

"After I had been there about half a year and developed a close rapport with Meng, he confided to me that Zhen Wu had appeared to him in a revelatory dream and told him to move to the States and there ensure survival of Taoist sciences until the time was right for their return to China: also, to develop the ancient Taoist knowledge into a modern science of life, available to people of all national backgrounds. We are working on all that right now. Our computer network is growing steadily and we are collecting some amazing information from all over the world. I can show you some of this when we arrive. The agricultural experiments are progressing well, though we have a lot to learn about cold weather, high-altitude food production. And we are beginning to build some good roots in the community. Though at first the locals considered us 'weird,' we are now on very friendly terms, and their children visit us regularly to help with chores and learn some basic martial arts. Some of the older folks have come for herbal healing work or acupuncture treatments. People from other places are starting to hear about us and visit occasionally. Meng does not want any 'advertising,' simply to practice our own Tao and let things grow in an organic way."

Even Peter had not been fully aware of the scope of activities at Purple Cloud Mountain. As we traveled on, he and I exchanged news and stories of recent events. He was still as energetic as ever and immersed in numerous scholarly and artistic pursuits of his own, while working part-time as assistant curator of the Asian Collection at Boston's Museum of Fine Arts. We rode further in silence and I dozed off, somewhat fatigued by the long journey from the west.

As late afternoon painted the treetops and mountain summits with its golden roseate hue, we arrived at Purple Cloud. Nestled into a beautiful setting, in perfect conformity with the principles of Feng Shui, the community was quite a surprise. I had expected to see an old New England farmstead and perhaps some gardens, but here was a large solar greenhouse, wind-powered electrical generating system, a fish pond partially concealed under snow, and a satellite dish antenna! Despite the modern accouterments, the place fairly breathed peace and enchantment. The dark grove of conifers to the hilly north gave shelter from the most arctic winds, and there was a wide open expanse and two ponds on the southern side. The lingering sun of winter's afternoon, the delicate light, and the visual balance between all the elements gave the entire area a feeling of deep harmony and fittingness.

When we drove up the driveway, two beautiful little girls ran out to greet us with happy smiles. They were Roger's daughters. As we alighted from the car and Roger stooped to hug and pick up each daughter, a stalwart elder gentleman emerged from the white farmhouse and slowly approached. Rosy cheeked, with long white hair but no topknot, he walked erect and with a balanced, powerful, measured stride. It was immediately apparent to any practiced eye that here was a martial artist in the old tradition; his very presence emanated "martial virtue." Though his power and energy were obvious, what struck me even more was his state of apparent happiness and simplicity. There seemed nothing affected about him; his bearing exuded a sort of twinkling energy and his eyes were extraordinarily bright. Though it was obvious that he had years, indeed decades, of cultivation behind him, all of that was now manifest as a quiet palpable happiness and almost childlike simplicity.

"Welcome, dear Tao-brother, and friend of Purple-Gold! It is wonderful that you are here. I always knew that somehow Fate would allow us to meet in this lifetime." He took my arm and looked deeply into my eyes. "Please come in for tea; we have much to talk about." The large living room was warm with a cheery fire in the fireplace. Peter lit his pipe and just sat smiling to himself, while Roger entered with the girls in tow. In a few moments Meng emerged from the kitchen with a large teapot in one hand and cider bottle in the other. The girls opted for cider and we sat down to the ritual pot of tea that gives people time to entrain and is obligatory for Chinese before any business or serious conversation can be carried on.

While the girls chatted on about their daily activities, and Peter sat puffing with a contemplative air, I told Meng about my meetings with Purple-Gold and Hollow Valley, my return to the States, and recent activities in the West. He listened with calm attentiveness. After a short time, a young Chinese woman appeared to announce that supper was ready and we repaired to the ample kitchen. While we had been talking, I had smelled delicious aromas wafting from behind the closed kitchen door, but I was quite unprepared for this lavish feast. A full twelve course ceremonial dinner was served in traditional Chinese style. The young woman was Meng's daughter-in-law and as she proffered each dish, she apologized for its lack of taste and for her own inabilities as a cook. We had to coax her to bring each dish to the table. Of course everything was superlative and I learned that she had once run a very fashionable restaurant in Shanghai.

After a leisurely dinner, followed by some fragrant tea and a bit more light conversation, Meng announced that it was nearing his bedtime, and retired. "He meditates for several hours each evening,"

Roger told me, "and though it is not really late, tomorrow will be a very full day so we might as well get a good night's rest." Roger withdrew, while Peter and I talked on till far into the night. Then we too retired.

The sound of a soft yet penetrating gong awakened me from a refreshing and deep sleep. Dressing quickly, I went down the hallway toward the faint aroma of fine incense. It was barely light, but the waning planets and gentle gold luster from the East presaged a clear day. Roger beckoned me into a small room on the west side of the house, where the light was still very subdued. Candles were alight and the "pine wind" incense set a mood of winter solitude and austerity. Meng was seated in the center, facing a small altar with images of Shou Lao and Zhen Wu, God of the Polestar and patron of Wu Dang Mountain. Peter and Meng's daughter-in-law were also there, as was a younger Chinese man whom I assumed to be Meng's son. After we had gotten settled, Meng chanted a few sutras to Zhen Wu; then we each circulated the Light in our own way. Upon opening our eyes, the room was already bright and we rose slowly from our sitting cushions and stretched. Now Meng's rosy glow was even more intense than the evening before. The positive energy in the room was palpable and thoroughly enlivened our *qi* and spirits.

After making sure that we were well padded, we went to the chilly outdoors, where the air was frosty, but genial, and there was no wind. For the next half hour we practiced a form of warming *qigong* that I had never seen before. Peter and I followed the others through their movements and breath patterns. The set was very opening and warming, preparing us well for Form practice. Entering a small barn, we found a beautiful studio with some photos of Wu Dang, statue of Zhang San Feng, and a rack with classical weapons. Thoroughly warmed by the *qigong*, we were able to remove the heaviest layers of outer clothing and practice very comfortably even though the studio was unheated. Meng went through the stately yet athletic movements of the rarely seen Wu Dang Taiji Quan, and then the Wu Dang solo Taiji Sword sets, accompanied by the younger Mengs and Roger. Peter, more devoted to the literary arts, practiced some of the famed Five Animal Frolics and I did a few of my own sets. An hour later we were all rubicund and energized, and well ready for a hearty meal.

Following a brief respite, we sat down to steaming bowls of congee with bits of chicken and vegetables, excellent to restore the body after practice, yet not congesting or overfilling. After breakfast we began the daily round of chores. Roger checked the greenhouse and did some work at the computer; the girls tended the animals (goats, horses, and chickens); Peter, a gourmet, assisted Mrs. Meng in the kitchen, while Old Meng and I went out to the woodpile. The tang of wood smoke had spiced the air since the previous evening and now it was time to pay our dues for the warmth received. We took turns splitting and stacking. I expected him to be vigorous enough, but was astonished at his energy and endurance.

My long stay in the west had not helped my physical condition. Though I had done some Forms daily and continued inner cultivation, my professional activities had been so all encompassing that I had little time for outdoor physical work. Now it was with a considerable sense of embarrassment that I found myself unable to keep pace with an octogenarian on the splitting stumps. I noticed too, with great amazement, that it took him only one swing to split each piece. First he would center and breathe deeply, then align his body precisely with the piece of wood. When the maul descended, each piece was split clean through. "Who needs martial arts forms?" he grinned, "they are mostly entertainment anyway. Once one has developed *qi*, <u>any</u> activity can cultivate it further. Cutting vegetables, painting, or woodcutting—they differ only in externals. The concentration of internal energy is very similar and they are all means of developing *kung fu*. If I may say so, you could use more time at the wood pile. Your inner energy is quite strong and well centered, but lacks the crisp quality when discharged. It must be '*gan cui*' crisp and clean, with no 'fibers' remaining. If you stay here for a few months, I think we can give your martial arts some necessary finishing touches."

He spoke in perfect English, with only a slight British tinge. Around noon a younger Chinese appeared, whom Meng introduced as his son. Young Meng, a man in his early fifties, looked not more than thirty-five and was obviously quite strong. With a winning smile he invited us both to stop working and eat lunch.

After a delicious midday repast, while everyone else took a post-prandial siesta, young Meng told me his story. Miao Zhen was the eldest son and had been groomed to follow his father as a master physician and herbalist. He went to the finest schools and later apprenticed with the very best teachers. Becoming a well respected herbal master in his own right, he had a clientele of the elite Shanghai families and married the daughter of one of the wealthiest bankers. He had also studied martial arts since his youth and was well versed in several systems, specializing in Fujian White Crane. He had achieved considerable prowess in his own martial practice and was quite proud of his father's attainments. Nonetheless, when his father "retired," left his family, and went to study with Purple-Gold during his latter years, he was deeply angered and distressed.

A spirited young man, he went after his father a few months later and found him in Shandong. Breaking all rules of courtesy he accused Purple-Gold of violating the most sacred of relations — that between father and son and husband and wife, of breaking up families for his own personal ends. Touching his forehead to the ground (*ke tou*) in time honored custom, Miao Zhen begged his father to return to the family. Purple-Gold stood watching, peaceful and impassive. When the elder Meng reaffirmed that he was going to remain with his Teacher till the end, Miao Zhen abruptly turned to leave without farewell.

Purple-Gold called to him in a gentle voice and the two looked at each other for some time. Miao Zhen felt a remarkable stillness, power, and love emanating from the old recluse and his anger vanished. Approaching, Purple-Gold beckoned Miao Zhen to sit on a stone overlooking the sea. They talked for a short while and Purple-Gold taught him the initial purifying meditations for the circulation of the Golden Light. These exercises proved so startling in their positive effects that within a year of his return from Shandong, Miao Zhen had become a devoted Taoist and student of the *Taoist Canon*. Maintaining his thriving medical practice, he began delving into the ancient texts on alchemy, geomancy, and other Taoist sciences. He became fascinated with the possibility of selecting the best of the Taoist scientific traditions, correlating them with Western discoveries, and creating a new planetary science, embracing the best of the ancient and modern.

Though he had always been energetic as a result of healthy living habits and his martial arts training, the profound effects of the meditations surpassed his expectations. He imagined their immense potential for the health and happiness of people everywhere. He was sure he could adapt the essence of Taoist wisdom into a form that was relevant for modern needs and lifestyles, without violating its essential principles.

After Purple-Gold's death, the elder Meng had returned to the family, where he lived peacefully and harmoniously until the death of his wife. Only then did he reveal to Miao Zhen his revelatory dream of going to the States and establishing a Taoist center. Inspired by their sharing of a common dream and challenged by the great adventures to come, they resolved to preserve and develop their sacred traditions in a new land.

Following Miao Zhen's story, I went out in the crisp chill of mid-afternoon to find Meng again at the wood pile. We worked in silence until slightly after sunset. Entering the house, I expected to be tantalized by the aromas of another Chinese banquet, but instead the area near the kitchen was redolent with broiled fish and baking squash. Peter was bending over the stove cooking while Mrs. Meng and Roger's daughters assisted. "No one loves Chinese food better than I," he smiled, "Red-cooked duck, Mongolian lamb, 'drunken prawns,' and occasionally even bear's paw and camel's hump. But this is New England and tonight we shall follow our local Tao." Soon we were seated around the table feasting on delicious Haddock casserole, baked butternut squash, and fresh greenhouse vegetables. Apple pie with a morsel of sharp cheddar, accompanied by rich amaretto coffee, concluded the repast.

"We can't have the locals think of us as totally exotic," Peter beamed, "a good New England dinner now and then will keep us well attuned to the local vibes and feelings. Now, Meng Dao-Shih, I know that our special guest has been waiting patiently to hear your story, and I myself am still curious as to the details. Could you enlighten us as to the real meaning of your coming here and of your past adventures that brought you to this place?" The fire was emitting a deep, steady warmth, the aroma of tobacco and fine coffee hung in the air as Meng began his tale....

⟨⦂⟩⦂⟨⦂⟩⦂⟨⦂⟩

"As you probably know, I was the sixth generation of traditional physicians and my mother's family was very proud of our lineage.

"Naturally, from my earliest years I was groomed to take over the family medical practice and herbal business. My father, though a military man, was a great student of the Confucian classics who had immense respect for the old teachings. Seeing the inevitable trends and directions in modern Chinese society, he did not want me to have a military career, but hoped that I would embody the best of the old education and merge it with more modern ways of thought. Having grown up with the martial arts, he had great respect for physical culture and inner cultivation, and performed some stretching and *qigong* daily. In his later years he became less inclined toward vigorous physical activity, preferring the *wen* or cultural arts as his emphasis. In addition to his military expertise, he was a talented calligrapher and also became quite creditable in his playing of the *chin*. Still, he thought that I should have the best of physical cultivation in my youth, so at age thirteen he brought me to Mt. Wu Dang for Taoist training. Such training was not normally available to most youngsters, but because of his well-known and widely admired scholarship, and the long family history and influential connections, he was able to introduce me to the revered Abbot of Wu Dang, and so began my schooling in the Tao.

"I shall never forget my first ascent of that holy mountain. The thousands of stone steps, some already crumbling from the ravages of weather and millions of human footfalls, the ever-changing mountain vistas during the long climb, and the beauties of the Zi Xiao Temple and the Golden Pinnacle inspired me deeply. Most awesome, however, was the strange glow that seemed to surround Wu Dang. The air shone with a purple hue which emanated a powerful vibration. Even at midday the faint aura of purple surrounded the mountain, but it was most noticeable at dawn and dusk. I will always remember the luminance of the peaks opposite Wu Tang as they glowed through the 'purple mist', while we did our early morning training in the courtyard before the Zi Xiao Temple.

"It was the Golden Pinnacle, however, that was most majestic and awe-inspiring. After climbing to the very summit, over the famed Nine-Zigzag Path, I entered the Pinnacle Temple in which Zhen Wu, the Supreme Martial Deity of the Mysterious North sits enthroned, and below him Zhang San Feng, Patriarch of Wu Dang. Going to the Golden Pinnacle never failed to leave a powerful physical effect. Whenever I visited there, I would feel my crown tingle and a rush of purple-gold light traverse to the *yin tang,* and thence into the Lesser Heavenly Cycle.

"Simply being there seemed to set the circulation going and I experienced this the very first time I entered the temple, at age thirteen before I had done any Taoist practices whatsoever. I now understand why the old tradition says that where one trains is every bit as important as what one trains. One goes to the holy peaks not only to meet the masters who dwell there, but equally important to absorb the sacred *ling qi* [spirit-energy] of those places. Each of the holy mountains has a very particular *ling qi* — Hua Shan, Wu Dang, Tai Shan, and Emei. Whether Taoist or Buddhist, each peak became a congregating place for devotees of the inner cultivation arts because of the emanations to be found there.

"Awakening at dawn, we first did an obeisance to the Polestar, luminous guardian and protector of Wu Dang; then did our stretching, *qigong*, and martial arts Forms. Each morning before practice, often in the pre-dawn twilight, we would scan the skies for planets and absorb their energies into our bodies before training. We also kept close watch over the Solar Terms and lunar phases. My Master's special emphasis was on following the processes of Nature and harmonizing with them to gather energy. Though martial arts were given their due, and we did a great deal of physical conditioning, the overall emphasis was on giving the apprentices awareness and attunement to the subtle energies of nature.

"The most important thing was to relax and open to the powers of Nature, and Tao, to allow the body to become fully <u>charged</u> by the cosmic energies. We would imbibe energies from the sun and moon, planets and stellar bodies; there were specific visualizations for each of these practices. My Master taught that the human body can be likened to a battery that must be charged to its full capacity. Being fully charged means that one has abundant vitality and perfect health; the internal energies are so strong that no harmful external influences can enter. We became resilient and strong, able to adapt to heat, cold, damp, and other outer conditions without detriment to our health.

"As you are doubtlessly aware, all states of disease in the body have their roots in insufficient fundamental energy or unbalanced flow. By learning to charge ourselves continually through good diet, use of tonic herbs, inhaling clear air, and absorbing the subtle essences of stars and planets, we ensure that our Upright Qi will always be abundant and flourishing. Moreover, once we have become fully charged, we can 'discharge' at will, either to heal others or in martial arts. We can use energy from the palms to heal either directly or from a distance, and in times of necessity, a powerful force can be issued from any area of the body to repel an attacker. At the most advanced stages physical contact is unnecessary—some high level masters can emanate energy from their eyes alone to disorient a would-be foe and render him helpless.

"One time at Wu Dang, a small group of visitors came to pay respects at the temples. One of them, a well-built middle aged man, after touring the holiest sites, began to ask the host priest about Wu Dang martial arts. The young host, in deference to tradition, claimed to be unable to answer such questions, and summoned one of the elder priests. The Elder and the younger man chatted for some time about training methods, martial arts styles, etc. Although the younger man observed all the amenities and courtesies, we felt there was something sinister about him; a kind of dark aura hovered over him.

"Suddenly, without warning, he rose from the tea table and charged at the elder priest, who was quietly sipping tea only a few feet away. To our amazement, he came to an abrupt halt before reaching the Elder, almost as if he had struck an invisible wall. He stood unsteadily for a few moments with a look of absolute bewilderment on his face, before dropping to his knees, pressing his forehead on the ground, and apologizing to the Elder. The Elder smiled quietly, then arose and returned to the temple, remarking that he hoped the younger man had learned a lesson and would be more sincere on his next visit. Later, when we asked the Elder to explain what had happened, he told us that he had sent his spirit-power through his eyes and this had blinded the young man whose darkened aura could not stand the intense radiance of spirit.

"Still, even abilities such as this fall short of the highest level. What really matters is to build and store enough energy so that one can 'lift off' smoothly and powerfully during our passage out of this world of form. This requires great vibrational speed and lightness of body and mind. When one leaves this dense 'world of dust' one enters a realm of great subtlety and refinement where vibrations are on a far higher frequency. In order to function to the fullest capacity in that realm, one must have a strong well-harmonized energy body that can accommodate itself to the higher energy states of the 'Beyond.'

"Most people are so weighted down with accumulated toxins, tensions, and unresolved thought-forms that they cannot lift off smoothly at the time of passage and this creates much suffering and dislocation when they reach the world of subtle form. So one of the foremost concerns of the Taoist is to remain firmly rooted in this realm while always seeing the much larger Universe of which our small 'dust ball' is only one minute speck. We realize that our 'game' here is only part of a much larger and wider game being played in many dimensions simultaneously. If our concerns remain centered only in this world, our energies will never develop sufficient speed and vibrancy to fully ascend and our energy bodies will hover around this plane of life, finally dissolving back into the earth itself, or gradually dissipating into the void like mists dissolving in the sunlight.

"When we are fully charged and energized, we resonate with the pulses of everything around us. Waterfalls, clouds, sunsets, birds on the wing—we feel each of these in ourselves and the ever-changing drama of Nature becomes a constant source of entertainment and delight. Up on Wu Dang there was no TV or movies! Also, the very experience of high energy levels in our organs, tissues, and bloodstream creates a <u>physical</u> sensation of deep warmth and joy, which in turn creates peaceful mental states and spiritual equanimity.

"As far as 'self-defense' is concerned, the paradox is that only when 'self' is forgotten can real self-defense occur. Otherwise the ideas of our body, mind, possessions, and fixations cause fears and tensions that restrict our deepest flow of movement and awareness. Our training had as its first objective developing our sensitivity to the subtle energies of Nature. We trained on mountain heights, in caves, forests, chasms, etc. so that we could sense different types and degrees of *qi*.

"Sometimes we were led blindfolded on long hikes and had to describe our surroundings at every part of the trip. After we had mastered our basic martial arts Forms, we would train blindfolded, or in the deep of night, so we could improve our tactile sensitivity and awareness of sounds. We would engage in pre-arranged and free sparring sets, both empty-handed and with weapons. Sometimes we would fence with razor-sharp swords in deep caverns where it was utterly dark. We avoided injury by using our subtle awareness of energies and by listening carefully to the <u>sound</u> of the sword's tip swishing through the air.

"There were numerous other ways in which we developed a refined sense of *qi*. Now and then the Master would take a small group of us down to the cities, where we would observe people to sense their *qi*. We would sit in parks, restaurants, and markets to watch people walking and engaging in their daily tasks, always asking ourselves what was their level of *qi*. We would also diagnose their organ condition by their gait, gestures, facial signs, and speech, so we could predict with an astonishing degree of accuracy their level of energy, endurance, and martial prowess. We could see which parts of their bodies were strong and which were vulnerable to attack.

"In all of these situations, we were trained to observe by becoming empty and receptive, relaxing our minds while focusing our energy bodies in one direction. We would center ourselves and let the other's energy body interact with our own, which would give unerringly accurate information. Full awareness of the inner energies and intent of others was the yin aspect of self-defense. As we relaxed even more deeply, however, the yang aspect began to manifest itself. We could experience the transmission of electrical impulses through our bodies that would enable us to move far more rapidly than mere muscular-mechanical movements. As soon as the mind would direct, the impulse shot through the relaxed sinews and connective tissues, forming itself into a stunning, whip-like attack.

"We found that in Wu Dang martial arts strength and speed came from complete relaxation of the bodily frame and unhindered electrical impulse from one body part to another. When we trained with the senior students, their touch would make us feel shocked rather than merely shaken or pushed. As our *qi* level intensified even more, we began to experience our *shen*, or the mysterious spiritual quality of high-level martial arts. We were able to sense a would-be opponent's intentions and thus to know his strikes or attacks before they appeared physically. If we were sufficiently relaxed and centered, we would move as soon as we felt the opponent's <u>intent</u>; a split second later the attack would materialize into the very space we had just vacated.

"Nowhere was this effect more striking than in swordplay. The sword, which best exemplifies the subtlety of yin/yang interplay, and is the master weapon of Taiji and the Wu Dang tradition, develops its own unique energy, joined to the *qi* of the wielder. One's own energy body extends into the sword, making it an electrically charged object. Often we would find it mysteriously drawn to a gap in our opponent's defenses, the moment his energy body or concentration would waver to even the slightest extent. Like lightning striking its target, the sword tip, positively charged, would be irresistibly drawn to the negative pole of the opponent's energy defect. Sometimes training in caves or in the depths of night we would see an eerie bluish glow surround the sword's tips and these glows interplay and discharge upon one another as the swordplay intensified.

"The strange and sinister 'Thunder Magic' sometimes used by other schools now made sense to me. At Wu Dang, however, we used the sword as an implement of internal cultivation, to refine our awareness of *qi* and concentration of spirit. The sword forms themselves, embodying the perfect balance of yin/yang, create a state of unique spiritual joy and peace in the performer. In my later life, when I had become a physician, I never neglected swordplay, even though I had little time to practice many of the other martial arts I had learned.

"One of the highlights of my entire training was a trip to visit Hollow Valley. I had nearly completed the initial stages of my education and was a fairly competent young martial artist. We went in company of one of the Wu Dang Elders and during our journey he told the story of Hollow Valley's earlier life.

"Brought up in a martial arts family, Xu (his earlier family name) had received the very best tutelage in both external and internal schools. At twenty years of age he was already a promising martial artist and by age thirty was well known throughout the Northeast. A specialist with staff and spear, he was also adept at timed strikes and had never lost a match. Frequently he would be called upon to demonstrate his skills at the houses of the noble and wealthy. His Form demonstrations impressed everyone with their dexterity, vigor, and power, but even more remarkable was his ability to defeat challengers from many other styles and specialties.

"Though still a young man, he met each challenge easily and 'his art never left him.' Soon he had a comfortable position as guard and teacher at a prince's mansion in old Beijing. He continued seeking martial arts teachers and studying assiduously and grew even more formidable as a boxer.

"One day an elderly Taoist priest came to visit the prince and young Xu was asked to demonstrate his skills with the spear. Though the demonstration was flawless, the Taoist was clearly unimpressed and casually remarked that the young man's '*kung fu*' was no more than superficial youthful vigor. At that, Xu became enraged and challenged the Taoist. The prince hastened to intervene, but the Taoist calmly rose from his seat and said simply, 'Come on.' Xu charged in, but was completely incapable of hitting the Taoist. Using the best of his foot and fist techniques, he found that it was like trying to penetrate an empty robe. He never felt his strikes land on anything more solid than thin air, or the outer edge of the Taoist's cloak. Frustrated, Xu pressed on his raging attack with all the power and skill he could muster, but striking the Taoist was like 'hitting at clouds or chasing the moon.' Never once did the Taoist use an offensive move until suddenly with a wind-swift foot sweep, he dumped young Xu solidly on the ground.

"In time-honored fashion Xu touched his forehead to the ground and begged to be accepted as the old Taoist's student, but the Taoist refused, saying that he was an old man who cared only to nurture his longevity during his final years. Gazing off into the distance, he stroked his beard with his first three fingers and thumb, then returned to converse with the prince.

"Xu immediately detected the Taoist's veiled message and appeared at his doorway the next morning at three AM. They spoke for several hours and by dawn Xu had decided to leave his post and become a follower of the Way. Not much was heard from him for several decades, when it became known that he was dwelling at Hollow Valley, living the simple life of a mountain hermit.

"The four of us, three 'young blades' and the Elder, arrived at Hollow Valley just before sunset and the place was bathed in a unique luminance, not unlike that of Wu Dang. The color, however, was different—more orange-rose than the violet hue of our mountain. The hermit was busy in his garden, but soon had tea ready and we engaged in polite conversation. I was still young then and burning to know some of his 'martial secrets,' but decorum would not allow substantive discussion this early on. Soon we had a light but satisfying dinner and afterwards retired to talk further.

"To my disappointment, he seemed most interested in expounding on the medicinal properties of certain plants—nothing about martial arts or even Taoist training. Finally our Elder asked him if he would reveal how he had decided to embark on the Way, and leave his position as the prince's bodyguard. My two companions and I had almost drifted off to sleep, but now sat up in rapt attention as Xu told his story...

'Yes, that afternoon and night with Cloudless, my revered Taoist mentor, was the turning point in my life and set me on a Path I have never for a moment regretted taking. When I was knocked down by that old man, all of my previous training as a martial artist seemed fruitless and foolish. Of what use to train assiduously for years, even decades, only to be toppled by a gray-beard? My ambition had been to become a supreme martial artist and to live my life in comfort practicing and teaching my skills in the noble palaces of the Old Capital. And I had made considerable progress in that direction, despite my relative youth.

'When I found that I could not even touch Cloudless, my faith in my skills and techniques was severely shaken, but even more so when I was soundly defeated in the blink of an eye. That night Cloudless convinced me that the path I had chosen could only result in increasing mental turmoil and a sad end. While young, I could count on my youthful vitality; and during middle age on my technical skill, but there must come a time when my mind would be forever preoccupied with anxiety. Would I still be a peerless martial artist at an advanced age? Would I be able to hold my own against determined youthful challengers?

'Having no literary attainments, I knew that only my martial prowess could give me any security or station in life. And it was immediately clear to me that at some point maintaining unbeatable martial prowess would itself become a burdensome duty rather than a source of energy and joy. While I had always aspired to be a consummate martial hero, I saw that the other side was the ever-present onus of having to "prove myself" at any time, and the inevitable anxiety that would bring. Cloudless offered me a chance to accompany him as an assistant and to learn the rudiments of harmonizing with the Way. His presence was so "soft," yet powerful, that I accepted immediately. Though I continued my martial arts practice for many years thereafter, my main focus became meditation and study of Nature. I learned horticulture, herbal medicine, and geomancy.

'Cloudless and I would closely observe the coursing clouds, meandering streams, and arrangement of hills, always seeking the subtle movements of qi that underlie all external appearances. As time went on, I saw that Nature in its entirety is an energy-flow of vast dimensions. The sweep of *tides, rivers, clouds, the patterns of growth in living creatures, and even the movement of Earth in its solar orbit, and of the entire Solar System in the Milky Way, is part of a gigantic ebbing and flowing of qi embodying tremendous, unbelievable power.*

' If we can tune into this power and absorb it into our own body and spirit, the need for 'self-defense' appears trivial and childish. Nature itself becomes our protector at all times. Study of Tao is to live in this ever-present power flow with simplicity, economy, and trust, always guarding Lao Tze's "Three Treasures." You trainees are still young, but I hope you can heed my words.'

⁙

"I sensed the truth and profundity of Hollow Valley's story, yet I was still disappointed. There must be <u>something</u> he could teach us that would directly benefit our martial training. I knew that someday I too might be inclined to follow the Way of the Sages, but for now I was a youthful martial artist who wanted to perfect my techniques and bring honor to the Wu Dang tradition. I fell asleep frustrated, hoping for something better in the morning.

"At first light I arose, expecting to find Hollow Valley doing some of his practices, perhaps some Forms. I thought that perhaps I could 'steal some of his secrets.' But he was nowhere around. Soon my companions awakened and we all practiced our morning routines on the ridge near Hollow Valley's small house. As first light touched the nearby peaks, Hollow Valley entered the clearing with a huge smile on his face, carrying a basket of plants.

" 'A special treat from the mountains,' he beamed, 'with these leaves I will make you a delicious brew which will invigorate you for your long homeward journey.'

"He busied himself in the kitchen for a little while; then returned with an antique clay pot full of steaming liquid that bore a subtle yet penetrating aroma. When poured into teacups, it was a beautiful golden infusion with delicate yet strong flavor, unlike any tea or herbal mixture I had yet tasted. We tried to steer the conversation to martial arts, but Hollow Valley deftly turned our queries aside and spoke only of the local plants, streams, and mountain paths. After tea and a light breakfast, we prepared to depart and I still felt a bitter disappointment.

"Suddenly a strange urge took hold of me and I decided to 'test' Hollow Valley right then and there. I hoped to bring no loss of face to the Elder or my brethren, but was not this also part of the time-hallowed tradition? Either I would discover that Hollow Valley's talk of the Tao-power-flow was an empty illusion or I would receive a martial arts lesson on the spot. Without warning I leaped at the hermit just as he was carrying the clay pot back into his hut. He spun round instantly, holding the clay pot behind him with one hand, perfectly balanced and protected. I attacked with full force, but he instantly neutralized my strikes and with a huge grin patted me lightly on the chest with his free hand. I felt as though a bolt of lightning had struck me and was catapulted across the small garden area.

" 'My, but you are a determined student,' he smiled. 'Just remember that youthful strength and speed have their limitations.'

"The Elder was close to furious as a Taoist can be, but Hollow Valley was utterly unruffled.

" 'Feels almost like old times again...first in Beijing, then in my many training sessions with Cloudless; and now here in my place of repose and retreat. Perhaps this worthless hermit will never find true peace after all. It must be my destiny.'

"The Elder was apologizing profusely, but Hollow Valley politely went on.

" 'No matter, you are all stalwart followers of the Way. If you are looking for some more "training" you could accompany me on some herb-gathering travels into the mountain wilderness. I have often had to neutralize tigers when my forays brought me into their territories. Though my martial skills have declined, sometimes absorbing a bit of "thunder power" really helps.'

"He entered his hut and when I had regained my composure, I hastened in to apologize. He accepted courteously and simply and soon thereafter we departed. That was my first 'great enlightenment' in martial arts and in life in general.

"I remained on Wu Dang for several more years, but in my late twenties my father summoned me back to the city. For a very short time I held a minor civil post, which my father felt was important as part of my development. I married and raised a family, to my father's great pleasure. Nearing forty, I turned to the study of medicine so I could take over the family practice. After a few years of painstaking study, I became a physician and also learned how to run my family's sizeable herbal business. Mostly, I was happy in Shanghai; I had all the blessings that one can expect in life and my health, rooted in my early years of training, remained vigorous, even though I had little time to practice martial arts. Nonetheless something was missing. The luminous mists of Wu Dang beckoned me still, as did the *qi* of the high mountains and the simple life. Though I was a very successful doctor and businessman, I remained inwardly unsatisfied and resolved to 'retire' from the world as soon as circumstances permitted.

"In my late fifties, my sons had grown up and my family was well provided for. I left the world of dust and went to dwell with Purple-Gold and his small band of intimates. You all know most of the remaining story. The simplicity and harmony of life with Purple-Gold affected me deeply and I felt fully at peace once again. But there was one more 'enlightenment' I received while there. A young Japanese Zen monk, whom we later named Wind Dragon, appeared on the scene and stayed with us for some time. Though Purple-Gold was very selective about the people he allowed to surround him, he took a liking to the young Japanese immediately and gave him the honor of becoming his personal attendant.

"Though Wind Dragon was not at all interested in Taoist methods of 'nurturing life,' he did sit in *zazen* for long periods each night. And he was always there with a ready smile when any daily task needed attending to and accepted each job or moment of daily life with the same cheerful equanimity. The neighboring children all loved him and when there were no pressing tasks, he would be seen walking with them down to the seashore or up the mountain paths. He particularly befriended one little deaf-mute boy. The black-robed shaven monk would take the little fellow by the hand and they would walk to the village and back to secure needed supplies.

"The little boy had a fragile radiance about him—beautiful sparkling eyes with just a hint of deep sadness. It was obvious that his natal *qi* was weak and unbalanced. Nonetheless, he was always bright and cheery around Wind Dragon and soon learned to carry water and wood, as well as assist with simple kitchen chores. Though the monk tried teaching him, the boy could not speak at all, but seemed to understand some elements of human speech. Each day the two of them would sit quietly, overlooking the sea, and the monk would recite his four Buddhist vows, beginning with '*Shu Jo Mu Hen Sei Gan Do...*' ["All beings, without number, I vow to lead to Enlightenment."] Then he would take the little boy back to the village for the night.

"Years later I learned that the boy had lived only to his late teens, before dying of tuberculosis. He had never learned to speak. But on his deathbed, surrounded by grieving relatives, a faint touch of rose suffused his sallow cheeks. To everyone's astonishment, he sat up and his eyes sparkled. '*Shu Jo Mu Hen Sei Gan Do...*' he said in a clear, though weak, voice; then he lay back down and passed away peacefully with a smiling face. Wind Dragon had that kind of charisma. He seemed altogether 'egoless,' and moved easily through all the vicissitudes of life. His special patron was Jizo, the Bodhisattva guardian of children, who also guides wandering souls through the Six Realms of existence.

"After Purple-Gold's passing, I hesitated about where to go next, unwilling to reenter the 'dusty world.' One day Wind Dragon took me aside, looked at me with an expression of utter kindness and love and said simply, 'If Tao is everywhere, why can't you find it at your old home?' That was my second great awakening. The next morning I left Shandong and returned to my family. Since then I have found that 'home life' is no impediment to practicing the Way. There is really no need for lengthy special practices each day. Once one has attained a good foundation in training, daily meditation and a few Forms to retain physical strength, agility, and energy flow are sufficient to remain fully charged and to grow in harmony with the Way. The most important quality is <u>mind state</u>, 'Embracing the One,' as Lao Tze called it, remaining calm and centered amidst changing conditions, never letting them disturb or discharge our energy body.

"Well, dear friends, I have talked on and on, boring you with my insignificant monologue. It is now time to rest and commune with Tao. Late night meditation is especially effective because the mysterious energies from the outer galaxies are then wafting over the earth and we can absorb them to develop unusual energies and insights. I am an old man and will soon be passing on to greater adventures. Like Chuang Tze I am ready to 'roam at ease through the Ten Thousand Changes.' In passing, I will regret nothing—the final result of my decades of training in Tao is only this: I am left with an unfathomable love of life and unabated amazement at its infinite power, depth, and variety. I am passionately grateful to have enjoyed this brief 'butterfly's dream.' "

The fire had died down to softly glowing embers and the scent of Peter's tobacco was still redolent in the cooling room. We sat silently for a few moments; then retired. After a deep and refreshing sleep I awakened to see a light coating of freshly fallen snow crystals glistening in the rosy glow of dawn. The outdoor air was frigid and crisp; deep winter silence pervaded the valley and hill. I looked forward to enjoying some time in the mountains and wondered if I would ever want to return.

Chapter 17

Lists of Forms

This section is self-explanatory with lists of the Five Animal Frolics, long and short Taiji Quan Forms, Two-Person Set, and weapons forms for advanced students. The "Wu Ming Short Form" was created while I was living and teaching at the Wu Ming Valley House, hence its name. These exercises and Forms are practiced by my students at my Academy, according to their individual desires and needs. I hope these lists will also show readers some of the scope and breadth of Taiji practices.

Specific instructional DVD's on these exercises, Taiji Quan Forms and Weapon Forms can be found at www.totaltaichi.com.

Five Animal Frolics

The Crane:

- Crane breathing
- Crane's beak
- Crane spreads both wings
- Crane squat
- Crane stands on one leg
- Crane spreads wings behind
- Crane Walk: arms forward and push back palms
- Crane Walk: arms open sideways and return to *dan tian* ("Crane Prepares to Soar Aloft")
- Crane Walk: arms open sideways and press behind
- Crane walks along the river bank, spreading wings forward and back
- A variation with raised knee
- Flying Crane

The Bear:

- Bear turns (twists)
- Bear pushes behind
- Bear pushes down
- Bear puts out claws
- Bear double push with palms
- Bear double push to ground (bending forward side to side)
- Bear double push to ground (sit back as you push out)
- Bear walk: (Bear ambles through woods)
- Bear Walk: with fists
- Bear Walk: pointing at the Sun, holding up the Moon
- Bear Walk: plucking berries

The Monkey:

- Monkey grasping branch (holding and pulling)
- Monkey looks behind

- Monkey offers fruit
- Palms extended forward
- Fingers widely opened in front of chin
- Monkey offers fruit twice

The Deer:

- Deer standing
- Deer walks through woods (turns head)
- Deer turns head behind (palm to *dan tian*)
- Deer stretches down
- Stag leaps up
- Wild stag twists and sits
- Deer parts the grasses

The Tiger:

- Tiger searches for food
- Tiger seizes prey
- Tiger leaps from den
- Tiger leaps from den twice
- Wild Tiger roams the Steppes
-

108 Forms Yang Style Taiji Quan

Before Movement, There is The Wu Ji Posture

Section I

- Taiji Quan Beginning Form (NORTH)
- Warding Off—Left Side (NORTH)
- Grasping Sparrow's Tail, includes the four basic moves of Ward Off, Rollback, Press, and Push. (EAST, NORTHEAST)
- Single Whip (WEST)
- Raise Hands and Step Up (NORTH)
- White Crane Spreads (Cools) Its Wings (WEST)
- Brush Knee and Twist Step—Left (WEST)
- Play the Lute (WEST)
- Brush Knee and Twist Step—Left (WEST)
- Brush Knee and Twist—Right (WEST)
- Brush Knee and Twist—Left (WEST)
- Play the Lute (WEST)
- Brush Knee and Twist—Left (WEST)
- Step Forward, Deflect, Parry, and Punch (NORTHWEST, WEST)
- Apparent Closing Up (Withdraw and Push) WEST)
- Cross Hands (NORTH)

Section II

- Carry Tiger, Return to the Mountain (SOUTHEAST)
- Grasping Sparrow's Tail (SOUTHEAST); this time omits the Ward Off.
- Oblique Single Whip (NORTHWEST)
- Fist Under Elbow (WEST)
- Step Back and Repulse Monkey—Right (WEST)
- Step Back and Repulse Monkey—Left (WEST)
- Step Back and Repulse Monkey—Right (WEST)
- Step Back and Repulse Monkey—Left (WEST)

- Step Back and Repulse Monkey—Right (WEST)
- Peng Bird Extends Wings (NORTHEAST)
- Raise Hands and Step Up (NORTH)
- White Crane Spreads Wings (WEST)
- Brush Knee and Twist—Left (WEST)
- Needle at Sea Bottom (WEST)
- Fan Through the Back (WEST)
- Turn Body, Throw (chop with) Fist (EAST)
- Step Forward, Deflect, Parry, and Punch (EAST)
- Step Up, Grasp the Sparrow's Tail (EAST)
- Single Whip (WEST)
- Wave Hands Like Clouds (NORTHWEST, NORTH, NORTHEAST) 5 Repetitions
- Single Whip (WEST)
- High Pat the Horse (WEST)
- "Separate" the Right Foot (i.e. kick with toe) (WEST NORTHWEST)
- "Separate" the Left Foot (WEST SOUTHWEST)
- Turn Body and Kick with Heel (SOUTHEAST) Kick to East.
- Brush Knee and Twist—Left (EAST)
- Brush Knee and Twist—Right (EAST)
- Step Forward and Punch Downward (EAST)
- Turn Body and Throw Fist (WEST)
- Step Forward, Deflect, Parry, Punch (NORTHWEST, WEST)
- Kick Upward with Right Foot (WEST NORTHWEST)
- Beat the Tiger—Left (SOUTH), Stance to SOUTHEAST
- Beat the Tiger—Right (WEST) Stance to NORTHWEST
- Turn Body, Kick with Right Heel (SOUTHWEST)
- Twin Peaks Pierce the Ears (WEST)
- Kick with Left Heel (NORTHWEST)
- Spin Body, Kick with Right Heel (SOUTHWEST)
- Step Forward, Deflect, Parry, Punch (NORTHWEST WEST)
- Apparent Closing Up (WEST)
- Cross Hands (NORTH)

Section III

- Carry Tiger, Return to the Mountain (SOUTHEAST)
- Grasping Sparrow's Tail (as in #18)
- "Horizontal" Single Whip (NORTH)
- Wild Horse Tosses Mane—Right (EAST)
- Wild Horse Tosses Mane—Left (EAST)
- Wild Horse Tosses Mane—Right (EAST)
- Ward Off, Left side (NORTH)
- Grasping Sparrow's Tail (as in #3)
- Single Whip (WEST)
- Jade Maiden Threading the Shuttle—(NORTHEAST) right side
- Jade Maiden (NORTHWEST) left
- Jade Maiden (SOUTHWEST) right
- Jade Maiden (SOUTHEAST) left
- Ward Off Left (NORTH)
- Grasping Sparrow's Tail
- Single Whip (WEST)
- Wave Hands Like Clouds (NORTHWEST, NORTH, NORTHEAST) 3 Repetitions
- Single Whip (WEST)
- Lower the body like a Coiling Snake (NORTHWEST)
- Golden Cock Stands on One Leg—Left (WEST)
- Golden Cock Stands on One Leg—Right (WEST)
- Step Back and Repulse Monkey—Right (WEST)
- Step Back and Repulse Monkey—Left (WEST)
- Step Back and Repulse Monkey—Right (WEST)
- Peng Bird Extends Wings (NORTHEAST)
- Raise Hands and Step Up (NORTH)
- White Crane Spreads Wings (WEST)
- Brush Knee and Twist—Left (WEST)
- Needle at Sea Bottom (WEST)
- Fan Through the Back (WEST)
- Turn and White Snake Puts Out Tongue (EAST)
- Step Forward, Deflect, Parry, Punch (SOUTHEAST-EAST)
- Step Up, Grasp the Sparrow's Tail (EAST)
- Single Whip (WEST)

- Wave Hands Like Clouds (NORTHWEST, NORTH, NORTHEAST) 3 Repetitions
- Single Whip (WEST)
- High Pat the Horse (WEST)
- Left Piercing Hand (WEST)
- Turn Body Around, Kick with Right Heel (EAST)
- Deflect, Brush Knee, and Punch Center (EAST)
- Step Up, Grasp Sparrow's Tail (EAST)
- Single Whip (WEST)
- Lower the Body like a Coiling Snake (NORTHWEST)
- Step Up to Form the Seven Stars (of the Big Dipper)(WEST)
- Retreat, Ride the Tiger (WEST)
- Turn Body and Sweep the Lotus (WEST)
- Bend Bow, Shoot the Tiger (NORTHWEST, Punch WEST)
- Step Forward Obliquely, Chop with Fist (WEST, Chop NORTHWEST)
- Step Forward, Deflect, Parry, and Punch (NORTHWEST–WEST)
- Apparent Closing Up (WEST)
- Cross Hands (NORTH)
- Concluding Form of Taiji Quan (NORTH)

After Movement, Taiji returns to Wu Ji Posture, Undifferentiated Stillness.

After completing the entire Form, one should return to the exact location of the Beginning Form.

Directional indications refer to direction of the <u>center line</u> of the body.

Wu Ming Short Form of Yang Taijiquan

(Directions are same as in corresponding moves of the 108-Form).

- Preparation Form
- Taiji Quan Beginning Form
- Ward Off Left
- Grasping Sparrow's Tail
- Single Whip
- Raise Hands Step Up
- White Crane Spreads Wings
- Brush Knee Twist Step Left
- Play Lute
- Brush Knee Twist Left
- Step Forward, Deflect, Parry, and Punch
- Apparent Closing Up
- Cross Hands
- Carry Tiger, Return to Mountain
- Fist Under Elbow
- Step Back and Repulse Monkey—Right Side
- Repulse Monkey—Left
- Repulse Monkey—Right
- "Peng Bird" Extends Wings
- Raise Hands Step Up
- White Crane Spreads Wings
- Brush Knee Twist Left
- Needle at Sea Bottom
- Fan Through the Back
- Turn and Throw Fist
- Pull Back, Deflect, Parry, and Punch
- Grasp Sparrow's Tail
- Single Whip
- Wave Hands Like Clouds (3 turns to the West)
- Single Whip
- Snake Creeps Down (Lower the Body like a Coiling Snake)
- Golden Cock Stands on One Leg—Left

- Golden Cock Stands on One Leg—Right
- Separate Right Foot
- Separate Left Foot
- Turn and Kick with Heel
- Brush Knee Twist—Left
- Brush Knee Twist—Right
- Step Forward and Punch Downward
- Grasp Sparrow's Tail
- Single Whip
- Jade Maiden Threads Shuttle—Right
- Jade Maiden Threads Shuttle—Left
- Jade Maiden Threads Shuttle—Right
- Jade Maiden Threads Shuttle—Left
- Ward Off Left
- Grasp Sparrow's Tail
- Single Whip
- Wave Hands Like Clouds 3 Repetitions
- Single Whip
- Snake Creeps Down
- Step Up to Form Seven Stars (like the Big Dipper)
- Retreat Ride Tiger
- Turn Body and Sweep Lotus
- Bend Bow, Shoot the Tiger
- Step Obliquely and Chop
- Step Forward, Deflect, Parry, and Punch
- Apparent Closure
- Cross Hands
- Concluding Form of Taiji Quan

Taiji Two-Person Set (San Shou)

Divided into Parts 1 through 9

Each Part listed separately for Partners "A" and "B"

Part ONE (Yang Style Da Lu)

Side A Initiates

- Step Forward and Chop (1)
- Right Shoulder Strike (3)
- Long Rollback Right Side (5)
- Cross and Push (7)
- Left Shoulder Strike (9)
- Long Rollback Left (11)
- Cross and Push (13)
- Join Hands (15)

Side B

- Rollback (2)
- Right Slap (Split) (4)
- Right Shoulder Strike (6)
- Long Rollback Left (8)
- Left Slap (10)
- Left Shoulder Strike (12)
- Withdraw Body, Rollback, Join Hands (14)

Part TWO

Side B Initiates

- Step Forward and Punch (16)
- Hold Up and Shoulder Strike (18)
- Left Elbow Strike (20)
- Left Chop with Fist (22)
- Withdraw Step and Beat Tiger Left, Join Hands (24)

Side A

- Deflect and Chop (17)
- Beat Tiger Right (19)
- Push (Right Hand Leads) (21)
- Right Shoulder Strike (23)
- Right Chop With Fist, Join Hands (25)

Part THREE

Side B Initiates

- Press Elbow and Punch Face (26)
- Neutralize and Chop (28)
- Horizontal Split (30)
- Beat Tiger Right (32)
- Join Hands (34)

Side A

- Ward Off, Turn and Push Left (27)
- Deflect and Punch (29)
- Change Step, Wild Horse Tosses Mane Left (31)
- Turn Body, Withdraw Step, and Long Rollback Left, Join Hands (33)

Part FOUR (Eight Basic Move Da Lu)

Side A Initiates

- Pull (35)
- Split (37)
- Right Elbow Strike (39)
- Right Shoulder Strike (41)
- Neutralize and Join Hands (43)

- Ward Off Right (45)
- Long Rollback Right (47)
- Push (49)

- Neutralize and Press (51)
- Join Hands (53)

Side B

- Ward Off Right (36)
- Long rollback Right (38)
- Push (40)
- Press, Join Hands (42)
- Pull (44)
- Split (46)
- Right Elbow Strike (48)
- Right Shoulder Strike (50)
- Neutralize and Join Hands (52)

Part FIVE

Side B Initiates

- Step Forward and Left Shoulder Strike (54)
- Separate Hands, Control, and Kick with Sole (56)
- Neutralize and Horizontal Split (58)
- Left Neutralize and Right Chop (60)
- Step Forward and Left Shoulder Strike (62)
- Turn Body and Reverse Hammer (64)
- Neutralize and Double Push (66)
- Neutralize, Turn and Push Left (68)
- Withdraw Elbow, and Push (70)
- Squat Down to Neutralize and Push (72)
- Push (74)
- Join Hands (76)

Side A

- Turn Body and Push (55)
- Brush Knee and Punch Groin (57)
- Change Step and Jade Maiden Right (59)
- White Crane Spreads Wings and Left Kick to Knee (61)

- Step Back to Left and Hammer (63)
- Twin Peaks Pierce Ears (65)
- Neutralize Left and Punch Right (67)
- Split Elbow (69)
- Separate Opponent's Arms and Right Slap (71)
- Neutralize, Control Left Arm, and Right Elbow Strike (73)
- Fold and Chop Right, Join Hands (75)

Part VI Push Hands with Fixed Steps

Side A Initiates

- Step Forward and Push (77)
- Press (79)

Side B

- Roll Back (78)
- Push (80)

- This is repeated for three Pushes, then "B" Changes, Steps Forward,
- And begin next series of four Pushes

Now Begins "Old Style" Active Step Push Hands

Side A Initiates

- Ward Off (81)
- Hands Circle Clockwise, Step Back Right (83)
- Circle Clockwise, Step Back Left (85)
- Clockwise and Back, Right Foot (87)
- Counterclockwise and Back, Left Foot (89)
- Counterclockwise and Back Right (91)
- Counterclockwise and Back Left Foot (Warding Off Right) (93)

Side B

- Hands Circle Counterclockwise and Step up with Left Foot (82)
- Circle Counterclockwise and Step Right Foot (84)
- Hands circle Counterclockwise and Forward Step with Left Foot (86)
- Hands Clockwise and Forward Right Foot (88)
- Clockwise and Forward Left Foot (90)
- Clockwise and forward Right Foot (92)

Part SEVEN

Side B Initiates

- Step Forward and Horizontal Split (94)
- Beat Tiger Right (96)
- Step Up and Left Shoulder Strike (98)
- Change Step, Separate Hands, and Right Shoulder Strike to Center (100)
- Circular Elbow Strike (102)
- Step Back and Pull Down (104)
- Step Back, Pull Down, Advance to Left Shoulder Strike (106)
- Turn Body, Change Step, and Separate Right Foot (108)
- Turn Body, Change Step, and Separate Left Foot (110)
- Change Hands and Right Shoulder Strike (112)
- Step Forward and Ward Off Left (114)
- Step Forward and Ward Off Right (116)
- Separate Hands and Chop Chest (118)
- Neutralize, High Pat the Horse, and Kick with Left Sole (120)
- Turn Body and Sweep the Lotus Right (122)
- Squatting Single Whip (124)
- Beat Tiger Left (126)
- Step Back and Repulse Monkey Right (128)
- Repulse Monkey Left (130)
- Repulse Monkey Right (132)
- Needle at Sea Bottom (134)

Side A

Part EIGHT ("Three Step Da Lu")

Side A Initiates

Side B

- Step Forward Right, Elbow and Shoulder Strike (142)
- Ward Off, Turn Body. Pull and Split (Long Rollback) (144)
- Slap (146)
- Join Hands (148)

This series (Part 8) can be repeated cyclically, over and over, as a separate Da Lu.

Part NINE

Side A Initiates

- Step Forward and Choke (149)
- Turn Body, Rollback, and Raise Hands (151)
- Retreat to Ride Tiger (153)
- Cross Hands (155)
- Conclusion of Two Person Set (157)

Side B

- Cross Hands, Carry Tiger Return to the Mountain (150)
- Step Forward to Raise Hands (152)
- Retreat to Ride Tiger (154)
- Cross Hands (156)

Sides A and B

Conclusion

Cane Form List

First Row

- Left coiling, Ward off to left, hit right.
- Withdraw right foot, parry to left
- Step up, block overhead
- Step forward, strike from right side
- Double forward step, "hang up left" and "split"
- Turn body, coil cane around head, split
- Cross step behind, hold, and chop
- Reverse body into Horse Stance and "heavy split"

Second Row

- Turn body left, hit obliquely upward
- Step forward, block overhead
- Left hang up, hit from right side
- Step forward, "hang up" and split
- Raise right leg, turn body and block downwards
- Horse stance, split to right
- Coil to left, cross step, strike underhand to right
- Horse stance, split to right

Third Row

- Spin left, coil cane round head, hit left
- Spin right, coil round the head, hit right
- Coil step, hit downward
- Step forward, coil round the head and hit from right side
- Withdraw right leg, strike rearward to knee
- Step forward, split
- Horse stance, stir up to left and split to right
- Use shaking energy.

Fourth Row

- Turn left, block or hit to corner.
- Swing right, block or hit to right
- Swing to left (180°), block or hit to left
- Turn right, block or hit to right
- Turn left, strike downward to left, parry upward
- Look right, strike downward to right, parry upward
- Coil to left, cross step, strike underhand to right
- Horse stance, split to right
- Conclusion
- Overhead strike forward and return cane to original position.

Yang Style Taiji Saber Form

(Single-Edged Broadsword)

- Beginning Form (NORTH)
- Step Up to Form Seven Stars (NORTH)
- Turn Left to Form Seven Stars (WEST)
- White Crane Cools (Spreads) Wings (WEST)
- Wind Rolls Up the Lotus Flower (WEST)
- Oblique Push Saber (NORTHWEST)
  "Open Window to Gaze at Moon"
- Left Underhand Cut (Saber to WEST; body to SOUTHWEST)
- Right Underhand Cut (NORTHWEST)
- Push Saber (WEST)
  "Open Window to Gaze at Moon"
- Jade Maiden Threads the Shuttle (Saber EAST; body NORTH)
- Push Saber Horizontally (EAST)
  "Lion Rolls Ball"
- Oblique Push Saber (SOUTHEAST)
  "Open Window to Gaze at the Moon"
- Turn Around, Revolve and Conceal Saber (WEST)
  "Great Snake from the Wild Regions Winds around the Body"
- Left "Shaving" Stroke (SOUTHWEST)
- Right "Fanning" Stroke (NORTHWEST)
- Push Saber (WEST)
  "Open Window to Gaze at the Moon"
- Turn Around and Conceal Saber
- Underhand Cut (EAST)
- Capturing Saber (EAST)
- Underhand Cut (EAST)
- Double Kick (SOUTHEAST)
- Retreat Step, Beat Tiger (body EAST; face SOUTHEAST)
- Stand on One Leg like a Mandarin Duck (SOUTHEAST)
- Turn around, Revolve and Conceal Saber (WEST)

"Great Snake from the Wild Regions Winds around the Body"

- Drift with the Current (WEST, SOUTHEAST, WEST, NORTHEAST)
- Turn Body and Conceal Saber (EAST)
- Step Up, Underhand Cut (EAST)
- Jump Forward and Chop with Saber (EAST)
- Powerful Stroke Splits Mt. Hua (Saber WEST, Body SOUTH)
- Pull in Saber, then Thrust (WEST)
- Reverse Body, Step Up, and Chop (WEST)
- Return Saber to Original Position (NORTH)
"Phoenix Returns to Nest"

Yang Style Taiji Sword Form

- Beginning Form (NORTH)
- Step Up, Join Sword Hand and Empty Hand (NORTH)
- The Immortal Points Out the Road (WEST)
- Three Rings Encircle the Moon (ends (WEST)
- Great Star of the Dipper (Chief Star of the Dipper, God of Literature) (WEST)
- Swallow Nips the Water (WEST)
- Intercept and Sweep
- Right Style (NORTHWEST)
- Left Style (WEST)
- Lesser Star of the Dipper (SOUTHWEST)
- Wasp Enters the Hive (SOUTHEAST)
- Nimble Cat Catches the Mouse (SOUTHEAST)
- Dragonfly Sips the Water (SOUTHEAST)
- Swallow Enters Nest
- Look SOUTHEAST
- Look NORTHWEST
- Finish to SOUTHEAST
- Phoenix Spreads Both Wings (NORTHWEST)
- The Whirlwind, Right Style
- Lesser Star of the dipper (SOUTHWEST)
- The Whirlwind, Left Style
- "Going Fishing" Posture (NORTHWEST)
- Sweep the Grass and Search for Snake
- Right Style (NORTHWEST)
- Left Style (SOUTHWEST)
- Right Style (WEST)
- Embrace the Moon ("Hold the Moon to One's Bosom") (Look WEST)
- Send the Bird up into the Grove (WEST)
- Black Dragon Wags Tail (WEST)
- Wind Rolls up the Lotus Leaf (WEST)
- Lion Shakes Head
- Right Style (EAST)
- Left Style (EAST)
- Right Style (EAST)

- The Tiger Holds its Head (EAST)
- Wild Horse Leaps over the Mountain Torrent (EAST)
- Reverse Body and Rein in the Horse (WEST)
- The Compass Needle (WEST)
- Face the Wind to Brush off the Dust
- Right Style (NORTHWEST)
- Left Style (SOUTHWEST)
- Right Style (WEST)
- Drift with the Current (EAST)
- The Meteor Chases the Moon (Look EAST)
- Skylark Flies Over the Waterfall (NORTH)
- Pull Away the Curtain (NORTH)
- Move Sword Like a Cartwheel, Left and Right
- Swallow Holds Mud in Mouth (NORTHEAST)
- Great Roc Spreads Wings (SOUTHWEST)
- Scoop Up the Moon from the Bottom of the Sea (Look EAST)
- Embrace the Moon (Look EAST)
- *Yaksha* (demon messenger) Searches the Sea (Look EAST low)
- Rhinoceros Gazes at the Moon (Look EAST)
- Shoot the Wild Goose (NORTHWEST)
- Green Dragon Puts out Claws (NORTHWEST)
- Phoenix Spreads Both Wings (SOUTHEAST)
- Low Stance and Intercept
- Right Style (Look SOUTHEAST)
- Left Style (Look NORTHWEST)
- Shoot the Wild Goose (SOUTHEAST)
- White Ape Offers Fruits (EAST)
- Falling Flowers (EAST)
- Jade Maiden Threads the Shuttle (NORTH)
- White Tiger Twists Tail (Look EAST)
- Carp Leaps over the Dragon Gate (EAST)
- Black Dragon Twists Pillar (Ends EAST)
- The Immortal Points Out the Road
- Look EAST
- Look WEST
- The Wind Sweeps the Plum Flower (Ends NORTH)
- Holding the Ceremonial Tablet (NORTH)
- Return Sword to Original Position (NORTH)

Suggested Readings

Since Taiji is about developing an attitude toward life as well as learning an "exercise form," some knowledge of its philosophical and cultural underpinnings will greatly enhance your study and understanding.

Since we live in a most "un-Taoist" culture, some reading of Taoist classics and other works will greatly enhance your feeling for Taiji and related practices. For it is the philosophy of life (the Taiji Master's "secret strategy") which is every bit as important to your development of health and longevity as are the exercises.

One essential supplementary "study" which you may enjoy is Chinese poetry ,which conveys more than anything else the spirit of China, and "Tao" of Taiji. Whitter Bynner's *The Jade Mountain* is a good place to start....*Chinese Poems* by Arthur Waley is also excellent.

Reading List for Taiji and Taoist Studies:

Taoism in General:

Lao Tze: *Tao Te Ching*, the best known Taoist classic, over 70 translations in English to date. My favorite is Arthur Waley's *The Way and Its Power*. It conveys excellently and with impeccable style the feeling for Lao Tze's timeless classic.

Wing Tsit Chan: *The Way of Lao Tze*, uses one of the Taoist commentaries, whereas most translators have used the Confucian commentaries.

Cheng and Gibbs: Lao Tze, *My Words Are Very Easy to Understand* Best translation to date with complete Chinese text and commentary by one of the great Taiji masters and scholars of this generation, and T.T. Liang's main Taiji Quan teacher.

This leaves about 67 other versions; take the one that speaks most deeply to your own heart and spirit.

Burton Watson, tr: ***Chuang Tze***, the best modern translation of the second great Taoist classic.

Lin Yu Tang, partial tr: ***The Wisdom of China and India***. Lin's style is especially racy and elegant. He has a very interesting translation of the ***Tao Te Ching***, as well as some of the ***Chuang Tze***

Lieh Tze: Another great Taoist writer, stories even zanier and crazier than Chuang Tze. Only one complete English version by A.C. Graham. See also the version by Eva Wong.

Huai Nan Tze: a Taoist prince, writing on inner cultivation, as well as statecraft and other matters translated as ***Tao the Great Luminant*** by Hughes.

James Legge, tr: ***The Texts of Taoism***, Victorian style and now quite dated, but has some interesting insights. Complete Lao Tze and Chuang Tze texts, as well as some ritual texts.

There are now some updated translations of the ***Tao Te Ching*** based on recently excavated manuscripts from the Ma Wang Dui tombs

Secondary Sources:

Works of John Blofeld, especially convey the Taoist attitude and spirit, so important to the study of Taiji—Entertaining style and easy reading.

Blofeld, John E.: ***Taoism, the Way to Immortality***, best for historical information.
   Taoist Mysteries and Magic, stories and personal experiences.
   Gateway to Wisdom, guidelines to Taoist and Buddhist practices.
   Beyond the Gods, some good stories of Taoist life in the late 1930's, based on Blofeld's personal encounters.

Holmes Welch: ***Taoism: the Parting of the Way***, interesting observations on the ***Tao Te Ching***, some good scholarly material, misses the point when it comes to Taoist practices.

Taiji Quan master Da Liu: ***The Tao of Longevity,
The Tao of Chinese Culture***

Peter Goullart: ***The Monastery on Jade Mountain.*** An out of print classic, sometimes available on Amazon. Fascinating account by a Russian scholar who is fatefully brought to a real Taoist monastery in the 1930's.

Bill Porter: ***Road to Heaven, Encounters with Chinese Hermits.*** An account of how Taoist and Buddhist hermits actually live in present-day China.

Deng Ming-Dao: ***Scholar Warrior.*** Excellent and detailed description of what Taoist training is really all about. Most books on Taoism on English are primarily philosophically oriented; ***Scholar Warrior*** is about practice.

I Ching

The central source book for all Chinese Philosophy and Science. Many English versions of varying quality.

Wilhelm/Baynes tr.: *I Ching.* The standard English translation now, but with many small defects. Rather heavy Confucian-Germanic tone, but still worthy of deep study.

Chu and Sherill: ***The Astrology of the I Ching***, contains a translation, somewhat more readable than Wilhelm, as well as numerological and astrological information.

R.L. Wing: ***The I Ching Workbook
The Illustrated I Ching***

The ***Workbook*** has more commentary, the ***Illustrated I Ching*** more art reproductions. Not a translation, but a paraphrase; still this may be the most understandable to those not already familiar with Chinese philosophy. Also probably the easiest text to use for first attempts at divination.

Hellmut Wilhelm: *Eight Lectures on the I Ching;*
    Heaven, Earth, and Man in the Book of
    Changes;
Lectures on the I Ching , Constancy and Change

Each of these three series of lectures on the *I Ching* is done with impeccable scholarship and insight. The books are unrivalled for providing interesting historical insights. Often understanding the historical allusions behind a certain Hexagram line's commentary will reveal a whole new vista of meaning.

Richard John Lynn: *The Classic of Changes, A New Translation of the I Ching as Interpreted by Wang Bi.*
This is a very good, traditional translation of the *I Ching*.
Wang Bi was the primary commentator on the *I* for many centuries and provided the Confucian framework from which the book was largely interpreted. (Wilhelm's translation is also from a Confucian standpoint).

Still, this is an accurate and readable version.

Alfred Huang: *The Complete I Ching.* Beautifully laid out and arranged. Very clear, epigrammatic translation. Excellent commentary.

Wu Jing-Nuan: *Yi Jing.* My own personal favorite. A "shamanic" translation, based on real scholarship. The ancient Diviners who put the *I Ching* together were not Confucian scholars. They were people of profound insight who could "divine" simply by looking at "oracle bones"—bones or later shells that were cracked by applying heat—or by observing objects of nature.

This version of the *I Ching* helps the reader to develop his/her own insight on the lines themselves.

Da Liu: *I Ching Numerology.* Fascinating book showing "alternate" ways to divine using the *I Ching.* Ways to get messages simply by looking at real-life events and interpreting them via the Trigrams.

Taiji Quan

T.T. Liang and Paul B. Gallagher (Editor): *T'ai Chi Ch'uan for Health and Self-Defense*, Random House Paperback. Complete translation of the major Taiji writings with excellent commentary, Taiji stories, and much more.

Sifu Ray Hayward: *T'ai Chi Ch'uan—Lessons with Master T.T. Liang.* Ray Hayward studied closely with Master Liang for over 20 years and took copious notes of all his training sessions. This remarkable book reveals some real "secrets" of the art, which you will not find in any other book. Profound principles many teachers don't even know about and most will never teach.

Sifu Ray Hayward (Editor): *String of Pearls.* Memorial volume on the tenth anniversary of his school in Minneapolis. Numerous essays by T.T. Liang, Sifu Hayward, and Paul Abdella (the two formally-designated Disciples of Liang), Master Wai Lun Choi, and students. Beautifully done with many photos, and the essays are superb. See www.tctaichi.com.

Jou Tsung Hua: *The Tao of Taiji Quan.* Excellent source book on all aspects of Taiji philosophy, history, and practice. Translations of Classics, stories, training guides. Not a "how-to" book for learning Form, but a very complete overview.

Cheng Man-Ching/Robert W. Smith: *T'ai Chi.* One of the earliest Western Taiji books, photos of the Master a valuable resource. Over priced, but well-produced text, now quite dated.

Cheng Man-Ching: *Thirteen Chapters*, translated by Prof. Doug Wile. Essays by Cheng from the 1950's, superb blend of Taoist philosophy, medicine, and Taiji.

Douglas Wile: ***T'ai Chi Touchstones, Yang Family Secret Transmissions.*** Ideal for the more advanced student, translations of essays by Yang style masters. Photos of Yang Ch'eng Fu demonstrating applications.

Douglas Wile: ***Lost T'ai Chi Classics from the Late Ch'ing Dynasty.*** A book for advanced students and scholars of Taiji Quan. Copious scholarly information on Taiji history, lineages, classic writings, etc. Classic writings printed in Chinese in the Appendix.

Scott Rodell: ***Taiji Notebook for Martial Artists.*** An excellent book on the martial training aspects of Taiji Quan—and why they are essential to gaining the health and meditative benefits of the art. See www.grtc.org

Ron Sieh: ***T'ai Chi Ch'uan, the Internal Tradition.*** A student of Peter Ralston, Sieh teaches how to learn Taiji Quan from the inside, by feeling, rather than as an external set of movements.

Trevor Carolan: ***Return to Stillness: Twenty Years with a Tai Chi Master.*** Evocative story of a student seeking and finding his "master." Beautifully written with a sincere and touching love for his teacher. Many valuable insights.

Yearing Chen: ***Taiji Quan, Its Effects and Practical Applications.*** One of the earliest and best complete source books. Partial translation of his complete compendium on all aspects of the Yang Style.

Yang Jwing-Ming: ***Yang Style Taiji Quan.*** Good source for applications, two-person set and sword techniques. More a "kung fu" sense of applications. See Professor Yang's other books on Taiji Applications, ***Classics***, etc.

Benjamin Lo/Martin Inn (tr). ***Cheng Tzu's Thirteen Treatises on T'ai Chi Ch'uan*** (North Atlantic Books, Berkeley). Same material as Douglas Wile's book, referenced above. Excellent photos of Professor Cheng in his heyday.

Kenneth Cohen: *The Way of Qigong.* By far the best general book on *qigong* in English. Impeccable scholarship, but very readable and informative in a broad range of topics: *qigong, neigong,* history and philosophy which underlies the practices.

See www.qigonghealing.com.

Fu Zhongwen, Louis Swain (tr.): *Mastering Yang Style Taijiquan* Excellent, fully illustrated translation of Yang Ch'eng Fu's *Yang Shih Taijiquan,* the standard-setting book on modern Yang Style Taiji Quan.

Sophia Delza: *T'ai Chi Ch'uan, Body and Mind in Harmony, The Integration of Meaning and Method.* For those interested only in the health and meditative benefits of Taiji, this is an interesting book. Much historical and philosophical information. Line drawings illustrating the "108" Wu Style Solo Form. Part Three of the book discusses at great length some of the principles summed up in Chapter 2 "Reflections" in this book.

Books on Chinese Philosophy

Arthur Waley: *Three Ways of Thought in Ancient China.* Taoist, Confucian, and Legalist Sections. Very good rendition of *Chuang Tze* excerpts.

James Legge, tr: *The Four Books.* The very heart of Confucian tradition. Although these books probably seem very quaint and "stuffy" today, I remember being at a lecture in which Cheng Man Ch'ing said the *Four Books* were absolutely essential for any Taiji student.

Ilza Veith, tr.: *Yellow Emperor's Book of Internal Medicine,* Partial and somewhat incorrect translation, but still worthwhile for its emphasis on <u>health cultivation</u> as way to union with Tao.

There are also a few more modern translations which you might want to look at.

Joseph Needham, Cambridge University, ed: ***Science and Civilization in China***, A grand work, far and away the best of its kind in English. Impeccable scholarship, superb notes with Chinese characters and titles. Volumes on Taoist alchemy are especially interesting (V, 2.3). Found in many large libraries.

Seven or Eight huge volumes dealing with every aspect of the topic.

Miscellaneous

Shunryu Suzuki: ***Zen Mind, Beginner's Mind***, advice about meditation and life by a wonderful and wise Zen master.

Whitter Bynner, ed.: ***The Jade Mountain***, Anthology of 300 famous Tang Dynasty poems. Excellent way to acquire the <u>feeling</u> and poetic sensibility to Nature of scholar officials in China's Golden Age. Translation's a bit "rosy", but still very good.

Arthur Waley, tr: ***Translations from the Chinese by Arthur Waley,*** More Chinese poetry, superbly translated.

Sun Tze (Griffiths tr): ***The Art of War***, Yin/Yang philosophy applied to military campaigns. Over 2000 years old, still widely studied by Chinese strategists.

There are now numerous translations of Sun Tze's great Classic. It applies Taiji strategy to military campaigns, but has a very broad applicability beyond warfare.

Ted Kaptchuk: ***The Web that Has No Weaver.*** Excellent survey of fundamental principles of Chinese medicine. Very complete and practical. Scholarly, yet very accessible.

Periodicals

T'ai Chi, edited by Marvin Smalheiser, excellent journal of Taiji happenings, with many articles and interviews with experienced masters and teachers. Must reading for all serious students. (Wayfarer Publications, P.O. Box 26156, Los Angeles, CA 90026)

Journal of Asian Martial Arts: often has excellent articles on Taiji Quan and other Chinese "internal Martial Arts."

Pa Kua Chang Newsletter: No longer being published, but if you can find any of these, they are very worthwhile. Real, substantive articles compared to many of the "fluff" or media-sensational articles in other martial arts publications.

Thoughts to Consider:

"Opening a book brings one benefit."—Old Chinese Proverb

"If you believe everything you read in books, better not read books."—T.T. Liang

Often, after a class, Master T.T. Liang would say good bye to a student, and then add, "Practice every day; do your best." I regret to say that for a long time I took that as simply a kind of "throwaway line"—-the sort of parting cliché one might expect a teacher to say. Many years later, I realized that that simple directive was in truth the very ESSENCE of lifetime progress in Taiji. And Master Liang was living proof until his peaceful passing at age 102.

PAUL B. GALLAGHER has been researching and practicing Chinese health arts for the past 40 years.

Paul is an advanced degree graduate of Harvard University, who then went on to study Taiji, Qigong, Chinese medicine, movement therapies, and philosophy with a number of eminent masters including Sophia Delza, T.T. Liang, B.P. Chan, Professor Kenneth Cohen, and Sifu Ray Hayward.

A Master Herbalist, Paul was also a founding faculty member of the prestigious New England School of Acupuncture near Boston.

He has written numerous articles, and edited *T'ai Chi Ch'uan for Health and Self-Defense* with Master T.T. Liang. (Published by Random House Vintage Series)

Paul has taught Taiji and Chinese health arts at Hampshire College, The University of Massachusetts, OMEGA Institute, Digital Equipment Corp., Pfifer Wellness Institute, and at many Taiji and internal arts studios across the U.S.

Paul was a Marketing Protege and Winners' circle Member with Marketing Genius Jay Abraham, and he completed the Excellence in Speaking Institute training with speaking trainer Ty Boyd.

In 1997, he started the Total T'ai Chi Center in Asheville, NC, where he taught Chinese life and health arts, as well as classes in achieving positive mental focus, realizing your dreams and goals, and savoring the ongoing process of Mastery—creating the life you'd really love to live. He is presently semi-retired from active teaching, but presents occasional seminars and coaches a few private students.

For information about books in progress, available audio and video programs, or scheduling a seminar in your area, contact:

Paul Gallagher
Total Tai Chi
POB 2352
Fairview, NC
28730

or e-Mail alltaiji@aol.com

24695484R00158

Printed in Great Britain
by Amazon